FOREWORD BY DR. SARAH MYHILL

THE CT3M HANDBOOK

Recovering Adrenal Health
using the
Circadian T3 Method

PAUL ROBINSON

The information provided in *THE CT3M HANDBOOK Recovering Adrenal Health Using The Circadian T3 Method* is for educational purposes only. This book is not meant to provide directions for the treatment of any individual. This book is not intended to replace the care by a qualified, licensed and competent medical professional. Care by a medical professional may be necessary to meet the unique needs of an individual patient. The author and publisher are clear that this book does not in <u>any</u> way represent the practice of medicine.

The author, publisher and others involved in the production and publication of this book do <u>not</u> recommend that readers alter their treatment that has been created for them by their own doctor or other health care professionals without individualised and clear guidance from these health care professionals.

Neither the author, publisher, nor any medical or health practitioners or researchers mentioned, nor any other parties involved in the preparation or publication of this book warrant that the information contained in this book is indicated, applicable, effective or safe in any individual case.

The author, publisher and others involved in the preparation or publication of this book disclaims any liability resulting directly or indirectly from the use of the information contained in this book. A qualified doctor should supervise in <u>all</u> matters relevant to physical or mental health.

Every effort has been made to make this book as complete and accurate as possible. However, there may be mistakes, both typographical and in content. Therefore, this book should be read as a record of the author's personal experience and <u>not</u> as a source of information on thyroid or any related health issues. Furthermore, this book contains information that is current only up to the date of publishing.

First published by Elephant in the Room Books 2013

ISBN: 978-0-9570993-2-6

In memory of Jeannine.

Acknowledgements

Jean Bassani, DC and Richard Herbold, DC - for their excellent contributions to the gut health and B vitamin information in Chapter 8 of this book.

Janie A. Bowthorpe - for realising that the Circadian T3 Method (CT3M) had far wider potential for helping thyroid patients than I myself had originally perceived.

The late Dr. John C. Lowe - for encouraging me so much to continue with this work. John, you are, and will always be, greatly missed. I will always miss you - your work and your friendship have meant so much to me, and still inspire me.

The Proofreaders - Susan Day, Paul R. Lundy, Alexandrina Smith and Julie White. Their great proofreading work and suggested improvements to this book have been invaluable to me. Thank you all so much!

Paul R. Lundy - who granted permission for me to include his article in Appendix C and who supported me in the editing stage of this book.

Lynn McGovern - who wrote Appendix D on adrenal issues and testing.

Dr. Sarah Myhill - I have admired Dr. Myhill's work with thyroid patients in the UK for a long time, and I am indebted to her for kindly agreeing to write the foreword for this book.

Thyroid Patients - Christel, Derek, Francis, Helen, Julie, Mary, Natalia and Sue who provided the patient experience stories discussed in the latter part of this book. To the thyroid patients who have generously shared their feedback on CT3M and my first book *Recovering with T3*. This feedback has been the driving force behind the creation of *The CT3M Handbook*. Thank you all!

The T3CM Patient Forum Administrators - Janie Bowthorpe, Francine Brown, Laura Hoey, Dave Kemerer, Bob Myers and Dawn Vo. The T3CM forum administrators have made great strides in understanding many of the health issues that can prevent CT3M from being effective. Their hard work and dedication to the health of thyroid patients is much appreciated.

The Very Friendly Staff at My Local Coffee Shop – including Mark and all the team. You guys kept me refilled with coffee and good spirits, as I sat there over several months, for hours a day, writing this book! I really appreciated the good environment, encouragement and great coffee!

Contents

Foreword

My patients tell me that they are increasingly being failed by their doctors, and nowhere is this more true than in the diagnosis and treatment of hypothyroidism (underactive thyroid).

Patients tell me that modern medical practice has been hi-jacked by the pharmaceutical industry, and that has reduced it to mindless algorithms, symptom suppressing drugs and tick box treatment regimes. The art of medicine, the desire to heal, the care for the individual patient is being constantly eroded. Doctors are more interested in tests than in patients because that allows for intellectually idle and emotionally devoid decisions. Consultation times can be cut short because all the tests are normal, and on the basis of this, patients are told nothing is wrong with them. Increasingly, I see patients disillusioned and dissatisfied because the root cause of their symptoms is not being addressed.

Many patients have worked this out for themselves already. Indeed I often tell my patients that their best doctor is themselves. The job of a doctor should be to recognise clinical pictures, point patients in the right direction, give them the rough rules of the game and provide them with the tests and tools of the trade to fashion their own recovery. The doctor's job is to do the coarse-tuning; it is up to the patient to fine-tune in such a way as to best suit their health and lifestyle.

This is where this book, *The CT3M Handbook*, is so valuable. It gives every thyroid patient the clues, the rules and most importantly the confidence to identify underlying impediments to recovering their health. It allows them to adjust their dosage of thyroid hormones to an individually tailored regime, in collaboration with an informed doctor. Paul's attention to detail is second to none. Indeed, Paul is listening to thyroid patients, making sense of their symptoms and signs in a way that is logical and with practical clinical application. He has turned himself into the attentive, caring, experienced and knowledgeable thyroid patient advocate that any patient would like to consult. Furthermore, he looks outside simple hormone issues to the many other dietary and lifestyle changes, which are so important for long-term health.

I would recommend this book to any patient with undiagnosed health problems or diagnosed hypothyroidism who has failed to respond to standard mono-therapy with thyroxine.

Dr. Sarah Myhill MB BS

Dr. Myhill MB BS currently works full time as a private GP specialising in allergy, nutritional & environmental (ecological) medicine. She has a special interest in treating chronic fatigue syndrome (CFS), has produced numerous publications and is the co-author of three original articles about mitochondrial dysfunction. Dr. Myhill manages her own practice near Llangunllo, in rural Wales.

SECTION 1

INTRODUCTORY INFORMATION

Chapter 1

Introduction

I am a thyroid patient who developed Hashimoto's thyroiditis soon after turning thirty years of age. At the time of writing this book I am now fifty-four, and have been living with thyroid disease for almost a quarter of a century.

Thyroid disease fundamentally changed my life. The reason for this is that the mainstream thyroid hormone replacement known as either T4 or *levothyroxine,* or by a brand name like Synthroid, did not correct my symptoms of hypothyroidism. I remained ill for many years, despite various doctors and endocrinologists reassuring me that my thyroid hormone levels were "normal" on this standard medical treatment. The conventional medication for hypothyroidism failed to give me my health back, and eventually I became a virtual invalid and lost the career that I loved.

I eventually managed to recover my health and get my life back through research, determination and trying other treatments. The critical part of my recovery involved the use of a currently rarely prescribed thyroid hormone, known most often by its simplified name: T3. The correct name of this naturally produced hormone is *triiodothyronine,* and its synthetic equivalent is known as *liothyronine.* T3 is the biologically active form of thyroid hormone. At the cellular level, it is the T3 thyroid hormone that keeps us well.

During the process of recovery, I learned how to use T3 thyroid medication properly and safely. Most doctors are taught that the only necessary thyroid hormone replacement is levothyroxine (synthetic T4), and they **never** prescribe T3. However, for some thyroid patients, T3 may be the only thyroid hormone that will enable them to regain their health. Many doctors also fear the use of T3 because they mistakenly believe it causes problems like high heart rate or osteoporosis. T3 can indeed cause problems, as can all thyroid hormones, but invariably any problems are caused by incorrect use. Another medical myth is that thyroid blood tests always reveal actual thyroid hormone activity. In reality, they merely measure the levels of thyroid hormones circulating in the bloodstream; they offer no insight into the actual effectiveness of these thyroid hormones inside our cells. It is such myths and the lack of a wider range of available thyroid hormone treatments that condemn thousands of thyroid patients to living a permanent hell with hypothyroidism.

T3 only treatment is sometimes required, as some problems can occur at the cellular level that other thyroid medications cannot correct. In my own case, T3 was my salvation.

More specifics on my thyroid problem and recovery

I was diagnosed with Hashimoto's thyroiditis at around thirty years of age. I was prescribed synthetic T4 thyroid medication and was told it would fix all of my symptoms. Yet the symptoms remained. I eventually reached a point in my illness when I had thyroid and adrenal issues. I had lost over one third of my body weight, and I was frequently passing out due to low blood pressure. I was virtually an invalid, sleeping for four to six hours in the daytime, as well as at night. I could barely walk around, and getting up the stairs was difficult. My career was lost, and in very many ways it was hard on my family.

During the first six years that I took T4 medication, my health continued to deteriorate. It did not correct my symptoms, however my TSH, FT4 and FT3 laboratory test results were improved and were all within the laboratory ranges. Eventually, T4 was stopped and I was allowed trials of natural desiccated thyroid medication. When this did not work, I was prescribed synthetic T4 together with synthetic T3. None of these alternative treatments corrected my symptoms either, even though my thyroid blood test levels all looked perfect. I remained with symptoms that included: exhaustion, weakness, dry skin, dry hair and digestive system problems. My mind felt like it was in a mist. I could not think completely clearly and I had low blood pressure. At the start of my illness I had put on a lot of weight, but as partial adrenal insufficiency also developed, I began to lose weight, became weaker and began passing out.

I was eventually prescribed T3 only, and then I began to get well. However, it took me three years to begin to know how to use T3 correctly. In total, it took me about 10 years to recover from the start of my hypothyroidism. I lost a decade of my life when my children were young. It then took me another 10 years to be able to reflect upon and communicate my experience with T3 in my book, *Recovering with T3*[1]. In *Recovering with T3*, I explain how T3 may be used safely, effectively and systematically. My background is in science and applied research. Because of my illness, I turned my attention completely to endocrinology and the understanding of how thyroid hormones actually work within the body. I used these investigations to work out how to recover from thyroid disease, and this work led to the writing of *Recovering with T3*.

I know that many patients feel well on synthetic T4. My concern is for the large number of patients who clearly do not feel well on T4 replacement. Sometimes thyroid medication that contains T3 is essential, even if thyroid hormone blood test results appear excellent when the patient is taking synthetic T4. This conclusion is very clear to me, both from my own experience and from communicating over the past six years with hundreds of thyroid patients from all over the world. Some issues cannot be seen through blood tests. This is because these issues occur deep within the cells of the body. In these cases, the biologically active thyroid hormone T3 needs to be present in sufficient levels in the bloodstream to allow enough T3 to become active in the cells. This necessary improvement in T3 levels can often be brought about by the use of natural desiccated thyroid (NDT), or by T3 replacement therapy.

INTRODUCTION

The adrenal glands and cortisol are central to this book

You will see that I am concerned with cortisol in this book. I found out myself that the right levels of cortisol were critical in my full recovery from hypothyroidism; thyroid hormones cannot function properly without a healthy level of cortisol being produced over twenty-four hours by the adrenal glands.

There are two adrenal glands. Each small adrenal gland, which is the size of a walnut, sits on top of each kidney. Aside from cortisol, the adrenals produce dozens of steroid hormones that are critical for good health. Consequently, maintaining the health of the adrenal glands, and allowing them to work as optimally as possible, is very important for general health.

Adrenaline, which is known as epinephrine in the USA, is the hormone that is produced in the 'fight or flight' response. It is the hormone that enables you to immediately cope with stress, anger and fear.

The adrenals also produce a lesser known (but incredibly important), hormone called aldosterone that controls the balance between sodium and potassium in the body. Aldosterone is also involved in regulating blood pressure.

Hormones called dehydroepiandrosterone (DHEA) and androstendione are made by the adrenal glands to help the body repair itself. Sex hormones are also produced to a certain extent in the adrenal glands, but not in the volumes secreted by the testes or the ovaries.

However, it is **cortisol** that I am most interested in within this book. Cortisol is produced in high volume by the adrenal glands, being part of a family of adrenal hormones known as glucocorticoids. Cortisol has several functions in the body. It can raise blood pressure, and also has a suppressive effect on the immune system by preventing the release of substances that cause inflammation. Cortisol is also important in fat, protein and carbohydrate metabolism. One of its main functions, though, is to raise the level of blood sugar by affecting glucose metabolism. Cortisol may be viewed as having the opposite effect to insulin. Insulin's role is to make our cells more receptive to the glucose that they need, and to facilitate the storage of excess blood glucose within the liver, muscles and fat tissues. Cortisol's role is to maintains a healthy level of glucose in the bloodstream. The adrenal glands produce more cortisol in times of intense stress, in order to protect us from the effects of this stress. It does this through its vital role in fuelling energy production and reducing inflammation.

To summarise, it is the maintenance of blood sugar levels, by a healthy level of cortisol, that I am most concerned with. It is due to this important function of cortisol that our bodies are able to make enough chemical energy within our cells to allow thyroid hormone to work correctly. I will discuss this in detail in Chapter 7 of this book. **However, it is important that the reader is aware that thyroid hormones will not work well in the presence of low cortisol levels and unhealthy adrenal gland performance.**

Thyroid blood test results on T3 treatment

I have used T3 only now for nearly fifteen years, supported by my family doctor and endocrinologist. Hashimoto's thyroiditis has destroyed my own thyroid gland. Consequently, the 55 micrograms of T3 I take per day, in three separate doses, produces rather strange thyroid blood test results even though I am perfectly well. My TSH is near 0 mU/L. My FT3 is between 8 and 9 nmol/L (top of my labs' range is around 6.5), and my FT4 is near 0 pmol/L. Most family doctors and endocrinologists would be extremely unhappy with these results and would say that I am hyperthyroid or even suffering from thyrotoxicosis, but I am not. At the cellular level my body is getting just the right amount of T3 I need, even though it is high in my bloodstream. This raises a fundamental point that is at the heart of many issues in thyroid treatment today. **Laboratory testing of thyroid hormones, and simplistic diagnostic work based on blood test results, is leaving many thyroid patients with chronic symptoms associated with hypothyroidism.**

In Appendix C there is an article written by my friend and fellow patient, Paul R. Lundy. In Paul's article, he outlines the historical 'development' of today's thyroid blood tests, and how they have come, mistakenly, to be relied upon in the diagnosis and treatment of thyroid disease.

In years gone by, thyroid patients would be examined and listened to by their doctors during the diagnosis phase of thyroid disease. Symptoms and signs would be reviewed in detail. If thyroid treatment began, then symptoms and signs would dictate whether the patient was correctly medicated with thyroid hormone or not. With the advent of thyroid blood tests, this has all changed. Laboratory test results now dictate whether a patient is deemed to have a thyroid problem, and these also control the level of medication that is provided. This is a flawed approach.

Paul's article highlights that:

- The laboratory testing reference range is NOT the normal range for an individual.
- A normal test result within laboratory reference range may NOT BE NORMAL for an individual.

Serum tests are only clues; they cannot tell us what is happening at the cellular level. **No laboratory test exists today that tells anyone how well thyroid hormone is acting within the cells at the cell nuclei and the mitochondria, i.e. the places where thyroid hormone actually works.** There simply is no viable 'one size fits all' approach. Each patient needs a solution that works best in their own body.

Consequently, we have thyroid patient forums on the Internet, patient websites, blogs, patient-written books, thyroid charities etc. By sharing the knowledge gained from our collective struggles to regain our lives, we help not only ourselves but others as well. Increasing one's knowledge is the key to a successful outcome and for becoming an effective advocate for ourselves with the health professionals with whom we work.

The above is the sad truth of where we are today. It is why I wrote *Recovering with T3* and why I have written this book.

The introduction of the Circadian T3 Method (CT3M) in Recovering with T3

The *Recovering with T3* book presents a safe, effective and systematic process for using the T3 thyroid hormone when other forms of thyroid hormone replacement have failed. This method covers basic diagnostic lab work, supplementation with important vitamins and minerals, and a detailed process that may be followed by a thyroid patient and their doctor during T3 replacement therapy.

Part of the T3 dosage management process introduced in *Recovering with T3* included a radically new protocol for using T3 and medications such as natural desiccated thyroid (NDT) that contain T3. I called this process the *Circadian T3 Method* (abbreviated to *CT3M)*. It is designed to help the adrenal glands function properly without the use of any adrenal steroids (like hydrocortisone), or adrenal glandulars.

I originally developed CT3M around fifteen years ago because even on T3 only replacement I still had adrenal symptoms. CT3M corrected my own adrenal function, and enabled the T3 I took during the daytime to work properly. I got my health back and in the process I discovered how to use T3 optimally. Many thyroid patients across the world are now using CT3M to recover their health after years of illness. Patients using NDT can also use CT3M, as this also contains T3 thyroid hormone.

During the many years that I was using CT3M myself I did not realise how applicable it might be to other thyroid patients. It is only since the release of the *Recovering with T3* book, and since many thyroid patients have used CT3M, that I have become aware that I should have communicated this technique far sooner.

I did not realise that CT3M would also work for thyroid patients using NDT. It has become clear that some patients can use CT3M with NDT for all of their thyroid medication, while others need T3. Some thyroid patients use T3 for CT3M, and NDT during the daytime. In addition to this, I had no idea that many thyroid patients who were already using adrenal glandulars or adrenal steroids, would be able to wean these alongside starting to use CT3M.

I have to credit Janie A. Bowthorpe for realising very quickly that CT3M had the potential for being more widely useful than I had previously thought.

It is now clear that for many thyroid patients, CT3M **should be the very first approach to treating any partial adrenal insufficiency** (which some people refer to as adrenal fatigue). Ideally, CT3M should be used before a thyroid patient considers the use of adrenal steroids or adrenal glandulars. It is also apparent that in some cases other health issues need to be addressed before thyroid hormone action and CT3M can be effective.

CT3M is not a standalone treatment for all cases of poor adrenal function, but it can be very effective when combined with a broader approach to health improvement.

A brief overview of CT3M

Many hormones follow a circadian rhythm with a pattern of secretion that is repeated every twenty-four hours. This is typically linked to our cycles of sleeping and waking, or daylight and night. Cortisol is secreted by the adrenal glands, with a steady rise in production during the last four hours of sleep. For someone who gets out of bed at 8:00 am, the highest level of cortisol production would occur between the hours of 4:00 am and 8:00 am. It is the rising level of cortisol that helps us wake up in the morning, with the highest level of cortisol in the bloodstream at around 8:00 am (for a typical person who gets up at 8:00 am). Cortisol levels then fall gradually over the course of the day, and are at their lowest between midnight and 4:00 am in the morning. The exact times may vary depending on when someone gets up in the morning (e.g. shift workers may experience a different circadian rhythm).

The Circadian T3 Method (CT3M) utilises the natural circadian action of the adrenal glands, and requires thyroid medication that contains pure T3 (so NDT may also be used). Once low adrenal function has been confirmed (ideally with a twenty-four hour adrenal saliva test), then CT3M may be used. CT3M may not provide any help if the thyroid patient has Addison's disease, or hypopituitarism, or an inflammatory condition that requires high doses of adrenal steroids (these conditions usually require lifetime treatment with adrenal steroids).

The basic idea behind CT3M is to address low levels of the active thyroid hormone (T3) in the adrenal glands, at the time when they are producing their highest volume of cortisol. CT3M can provide an 'adrenal boost'!

The CT3M process begins with the thyroid patient setting an alarm clock or mobile phone alarm at 1.5 hours before the normal time that they would get out of bed. A dose of T3 or NDT medication is taken at that time. The thyroid patient then goes back to sleep. By carefully varying the time (generally within the last four hours of sleep), and the size of this *circadian dose* of T3-containing thyroid medication, it is possible to significantly help the adrenal glands to produce more of their hormones, including cortisol. Cortisol is often low in thyroid patients.

Throughout the book, I call this early morning dose of thyroid medication the circadian dose. When circadian dose is referred to it means the T3 or NDT medication that is taken during the last four-hour period before someone gets out of bed in the morning.

Once this process begins to work and the adrenal glands begin to function better, the quality of sleep that follows this circadian dose is often far better than the thyroid patient has been used to experiencing.

In recent years, there has been research confirming that T3 thyroid hormone peaks in the body when the adrenal glands begin to work hard in the early hours of the morning.[2] These research findings support the ideas behind CT3M. The research basically says that after TSH has peaked each day around midnight, that FT3 also peaks some hours later.

So, the free T3 levels in a healthy person with a well functioning thyroid gland will peak in the early hours of the morning. This is normally not the case for those thyroid patients on any type of thyroid medication. This is because thyroid hormones will be at a low point in the early hours of the morning, and at a high point during the daytime – which is the exact opposite of how the human body is designed to work. CT3M aims to replicate nature by restoring a good level of T3 at the time when the adrenal glands begin to produce high levels of cortisol.

A large number of thyroid patients have used CT3M since the *Recovering with T3* book was published. Many of these patients had previously found that the only way they could cope was through the use of adrenal steroids, such as hydrocortisone or adrenal glandulars. When adrenal steroids are employed this causes the pituitary to demand less work from the adrenal glands. The consequence of this is often that the thyroid patient's adrenal glands become sluggish and less able to work on their own (there is concern that this may lead to long term issues with adrenal function in some cases). CT3M often works well enough to allow these patients to slowly reduce and then stop the use of all adrenal steroids.

Why is there a need for a handbook on CT3M?

When I first described CT3M in *Recovering with T3* I had no idea how relevant it was going to be. At that time I saw CT3M as a small part of the T3 dosage management process. However, CT3M is now frequently being used by many thyroid patients (who are taking T3 or NDT medication) to correct or improve the symptoms of partial adrenal insufficiency.

I have now received feedback from many thyroid patients who had suffered from partial adrenal insufficiency, and who have regained their health using CT3M. A few of these patients kindly sent in testimonials, and these may be found in the Success Stories section of my website.[3] Given that so many patients have achieved such success, CT3M ought to be one of the first treatment options used after low cortisol has been established.

Since the *Recovering with T3* book was published, vast amounts have been learned about the subtleties of using CT3M. Much of this learning is in the hands of the thyroid patients on many thyroid forums around the world, and is also documented on my own website.[3] It is also clear, given the success to-date of CT3M, that it will be in use for a very long time. It is therefore helpful to patients to have access to this up-to-date knowledge about CT3M in an easy-to-use handbook.

Since *Recovering with T3* was written, it has become increasingly apparent that other health issues may need to be corrected for thyroid hormone action (and therefore CT3M) to be effective. I discuss the need to combine the use of CT3M with a broader approach to health at various stages during this book. I also cover specific conditions that may need to be investigated and treated before CT3M might begin to work correctly. Having said that, *The CT3M Handbook* remains a handbook focused on CT3M. To make this book totally comprehensive, in terms of dealing fully with other relevant health issues, would be far too much work. It would also be beyond my capability to achieve, at least in a way in which I would be satisfied.

Goals of *The CT3M Handbook*

I set out with the following goals when I started to write *The CT3M Handbook*:

1. Clarify the Circadian T3 Method.
2. Answer as many of the important questions that have been raised by thyroid patients about CT3M.
3. Clarify the any unique situations and related factors that are relevant to CT3M, which *Recovering with T3* had no room to deal with, or that have surfaced since the introduction of *Recovering with T3*.
4. Keep it as clear, short and simple as possible, and without long descriptions.
5. Employ the use of **short chapters**, so that it is easily digestible in bite-sized chunks.
6. Make it shorter than *Recovering with T3*, so that it is quick to read and easy to use.
7. Ensure it complements *Recovering with T3* by only focusing on CT3M.
8. Focus on the practical experience gained from the use of CT3M rather than on medical research. I provided medical research references in *Recovering with T3,* and in keeping this handbook as short and as easy to use as possible, these are not repeated within this book.
9. Refer to information already covered in *Recovering with T3* within the text, so that readers may find the relevant section easily. Note: I have included references in the text, such as '[RWT3 6]', which via Appendix D will lead you to the relevant place within *Recovering with T3*.
10. Make it very clear that CT3M is not a **single technique** that will correct partial adrenal insufficiency in all cases. In some cases, CT3M will immediately correct adrenal issues and help individuals to recover very quickly. However, CT3M may need to be combined with the diagnosis and treatment of other important health conditions that are **impacting the health** of the thyroid patient.

The reader will have to decide if I have achieved these goals.

There remains a need for radical changes and there is always hope

The medical profession still largely ignores T3 and NDT thyroid hormone replacement, mainly due to lack of information. Very little appears to have changed in treatment practices during the nearly quarter of a century since I was first diagnosed with thyroid problems. The human cost of this slow progress is high. I have spent several years on Internet forums listening to the often heartbreaking stories of thyroid patients. Because of this, I am now far more aware of how thyroid disease affects the lives of many people. It is unacceptable – something has to change.

Most of these changes are straightforward, as the treatments already exist. CT3M is one such approach that works well for thyroid patients with adrenal issues. This is especially so if it is used before the thyroid patient has been exposed to adrenal steroid/adrenal glandular use for a prolonged period of time, and when combined with other approaches to healthcare. However, change is hard. The medical profession does not tend to look to patients for suggestions on what needs to change within diagnosis and treatment approaches. This is a tragedy. We know that huge numbers of thyroid patients are being left with severe symptoms of hypothyroidism or partial adrenal insufficiency due to rigid and ineffective treatment (often with T4 medication). It would be relatively simple for the medical profession to embrace the methods that we already know work well. Yet we wait for real change to occur.

However, I remain with some optimism. Some doctors have actually taken the concepts discussed within the *Recovering with T3* book on board and are applying them. Quite a number of these doctors are in the USA, but I hope that over time more doctors will begin to offer their thyroid patients a broader and more effective range of treatment options.

I would love to see the introduction of dedicated treatment centres within all countries. These could provide more in-depth support for thyroid patients for whom conventional T4 based treatment has failed. I believe that specialised centres would provide an interim solution for thyroid patients who currently feel abandoned by their own health care systems. Such patients are often forced as a last resort to attempt to manage their own treatment. The long-term solution is to make all the thyroid treatments available with proper support from health care providers all over the world, but we are still a million miles away from this.

Over the coming years I intend to make myself available to work with interested doctors, as I believe that long-term, sustainable change can only be achieved from within the medical profession. I would be happy to talk to any doctor who wishes to speak to me. My hope is that doctors and thyroid patients find the information within *Recovering with T3* and *The CT3M Handbook* of value. I also hope that my work with CT3M can play a small part in the revolution in treatment that thyroid patients so desperately need and deserve.

A few words of caution

I am **not** a doctor and have had no medical training. However, I am able to make logical deductions, perform systematic problem solving, and I can read and understand technical information.

The word 'patient' is used extensively throughout this book. I always mean that this is a 'thyroid patient', just as I have been a thyroid patient. I never mean that this is a patient of mine - because I have none.

This book was written in order to document the experience thyroid patients have had with CT3M. I hope that the medical profession will take some of this on board. I do not believe that this book can in any way replace the relationship between a patient and their doctor.

Any changes to a patient's medications or supplements should only be done under the supervision of the patient's own doctor, and with proper medical supervision thereafter.

I am not proposing that anyone applies any of the information, methods or suggestions contained within this book. A qualified doctor should supervise any course of treatment involving thyroid hormones, other hormones, prescription medicines, vitamins, minerals or food supplements. If anyone attempts to apply any of the information, methods, or suggestions described in this book, then I can take no responsibility for any consequences of this.

I am hoping that the medical profession will consider and investigate CT3M as one useful tool in an overall heath improvement approach for thyroid patients who have partial adrenal insufficiency.

Chapter 2

Circadian Rhythm and How CT3M Works

Cortisol is secreted by the adrenal glands in a circadian rhythm, with a steady rise in production during the last four hours of sleep. Therefore, for someone who gets up at 8:00 am in the morning, the highest volume of cortisol is produced between the hours of 4:00 am and 8:00 am. This circadian pattern of cortisol production is a well-documented medical fact. The exact times may vary depending on when someone gets up in the morning.

As mentioned in the introduction, a 2008 research study found that in healthy people free T3 levels in the bloodstream have a circadian rhythm, which is related to the cycles of TSH and T4.[1] This results in FT3 typically reaching a peak in the body around 4:00 am. A more recent study in 2012 found that the pulses of TSH are more frequent and also higher during the night.[2]

From the recent research, it is clear that TSH reaches peak levels in the body around midnight for most people. This rising force of TSH does two things in healthy people. Firstly, the high level of TSH around midnight drives the thyroid gland to produce high levels of thyroid hormones, which includes both T4 and T3. The high level of TSH also increases the conversion rate of FT4 to FT3. There are many studies that show how increased TSH results in a higher conversion rate of FT4 to FT3.[3, 4, 5]

All the cells in our body require the biologically active thyroid hormone, T3, to be present in high enough levels for the cells to work correctly. The adrenal gland cells are not unique, and they too require good levels of T3 in order to work correctly. As described in *Recovering with T3*, I discovered that by taking an early morning dose of thyroid medication that contains T3, the adrenal glands can be encouraged to improve their performance. In many cases this is enough to regain healthy adrenal gland function.[RWT3 6]

The Circadian T3 Method is an apt description of this technique as it utilises the natural circadian cycle of the adrenal glands, and it requires thyroid medication that contains pure T3 (not slow release). However, because it is a rather long description it is referred to as CT3M.

THYROID MEDS DON'T MIMIC HEALTHY 24-HOUR HORMONE LEVELS

I have just referred to scientific studies showing that TSH peaks around midnight for most people,, and that subsequently FT3 peaks in the body a few hours later - typically when the adrenal glands begin to work. These natural cycles apply to people who are healthy, have fully working thyroid glands and are not taking thyroid hormone medication.

When a thyroid patient takes thyroid medication, this natural cycle of thyroid hormone production will not be duplicated as precisely as it would have been when they were healthy and with a working thyroid gland.

Most people are advised to take their thyroid medication in the daytime. In the case of NDT or T3, the thyroid patient is often advised to take this medication in a small number of divided doses over the day. In this way, the benefit of increased T3 levels in the body can often be helpful for the patient, providing them with energy and a sense of well-being during the day. However, this usage of thyroid medication has some consequences that have largely been ignored by most of the medical profession.

There are several key points that are worth being aware of. Together, they make it more obvious why CT3M is helpful to some thyroid patients:

1. The use of NDT and T3 tends to increase FT3 levels slightly above the level that the thyroid patient would have had when their thyroid gland and body were working healthily in the past. In fact, many patients often do not feel well unless FT3 does rise to quite a high level with respect to the laboratory reference range for FT3. It is common to find thyroid patients who recover their health using NDT or T3, with FT3 levels near the upper quartile of the laboratory reference range for FT3, or even above this in some cases.

2. If FT3 levels are high in the reference range then this will tend to keep TSH either very low or suppressed. After prolonged hypothyroidism, TSH can also become maladjusted to a lower set point than when the thyroid patient was healthy in the past.[RWT3 7]

3. FT3 levels will tend to fall during the night. The reason for this is that the effect of the NDT or T3 wears off, on account of the short half-life of the T3 thyroid hormone.

4. In addition, for some thyroid patients, there will already have been a significant suppressive effect on TSH due to the daytime NDT or T3 medication.

5. Consequently, the production of T4 and T3 by the patient's thyroid gland during the night may be much lower than when they were completely healthy in the past. This last point assumes that the thyroid patient has some remaining healthy thyroid tissue.

6. Any reduction in thyroid hormone production by the thyroid gland during the night may be even more pronounced for those thyroid patients with greatly reduced thyroid function due to Hashimoto's thyroiditis, other forms of disease or atrophy of the thyroid gland.

7. It is known that TSH level affects the conversion rate of T4 to T3. If TSH is higher, the conversion rate is better and more FT3 is produced from FT4. If TSH is suppressed, the conversion rate is lower and less FT3 is available.[RWT3 8]

8. If TSH is lower during the night for a thyroid patient on thyroid medication (see point 2 and 4 above) than it used to be in the past when they were healthy, then there will be a lower rate of conversion of FT4 to FT3 during the night.

The consequence of all the observations in 1-8 above, is that for many patients who use NDT or T3 medications their FT3 may not be as high during the night as it was in the past (when they were healthy and without thyroid problems).

Prior to thyroid disease, when thyroid patients were in good health, it is likely that they would have been making far more thyroid hormone during the night and converting far more of it to T3.

This is not an argument against the use of thyroid medications like NDT and T3, because many people absolutely need them, and they are often far superior to synthetic T4 (levothyroxine). However, it illustrates that these medications do not mimic the natural cycles of thyroid hormone that are experienced when someone has a working thyroid gland and good health.

Thyroid patients using NDT, T3 (or even T4 thyroid medications) may well experience night levels of FT3 below the level that they experienced in the past when they were in good health. If FT3 is lower during the night, then <u>cortisol production</u> in the early hours of the morning may also be lower as a consequence. This creates a tendency for thyroid patients, who use thyroid medication according to the current medical guidelines, to be more likely to develop adrenal issues!

Thyroid patients (and their doctors) may not know any of the above, because night-time levels of thyroid hormones are never actually measured. However, the way the thyroid hormones and the endocrine system work leads to this possibility for thyroid patients. For some people with good health, and a lot of margin available in their hormone production, this situation may not be a problem. However, for others who are struggling, this may be a hugely significant factor.

Thyroid patients using synthetic T4 medications (like Synthroid, Levothyroxine or Levaxin) may also find that they have problems, as these medications are often used to replace the thyroid hormones of a failing thyroid gland. If the thyroid gland cannot produce healthy levels of T4 and T3 during the night, then thyroid patients on these medications may also find that they have lower FT3 levels than they had in the past. This goes a long way towards explaining why some thyroid patients using synthetic T4 often do better when they take their medication at bedtime. The reason being: this method is a little closer to a natural circadian pattern, although it is unlikely to make FT3 peak in the optimal and natural manner.

The above logic is therefore applicable to all <u>thyroid medication types</u>. Daytime replacement of thyroid medication has the potential to leave some

patients with <u>lower cortisol levels</u> than they had in the past. It may not happen to all patients; it will depend on how robust their systems are. But it could happen to some, and it goes a long way towards explaining why so many thyroid patients suffer with the symptoms of partial adrenal insufficiency.

DOES IT MATTER IF THYROID MEDICATIONS DON'T MIMIC A NATURAL CYCLE PERFECTLY?

The simple answer is that if the natural cycle of thyroid hormone production is not replicated, <u>some</u> thyroid patients will suffer, while <u>others will not</u>. Some thyroid patients, who have very healthy adrenal glands and few health issues, appear to be perfectly fine just using daytime NDT or T3. These patients appear to have good adrenal performance including good cortisol levels. Others do not appear to do so well, and have lower cortisol levels than they require.

Clearly, for people with chronic health issues, or compromised gut or immune systems, there is even more likelihood of less than optimal cortisol levels being achieved.

CT3M MIMICS HEALTHY THYROID HORMONE LEVELS

Thyroid patients on NDT or T3 medications will usually have high daytime thyroid hormone levels, and low or suppressed TSH levels.

In a healthy person, TSH rises and peaks around midnight, resulting in peak levels of FT3 a few hours later when the adrenals begin to produce high volumes of cortisol.

For a thyroid patient using NDT or T3, the normal circadian rhythm will be disrupted due to FT3 levels that peak in the daytime with low TSH levels. NDT and T3 thyroid hormone treatments will often result in lower FT3 levels in the night, which is due to a lack of medication taken during this night time period, and the effect of low or suppressed TSH. This is something that is usually completely overlooked by doctors and thyroid patients themselves.

Thyroid patients obviously have to replace their missing hormones, and they usually take them in the daytime. This results in peak levels of FT3 during the day, which is <u>not</u> what happens in a healthy person. Thyroid patients taking NDT or T3 in the daytime will tend to have lower FT3 levels during the night. Again, is <u>not</u> what happens in a healthy person.

The way in which thyroid medications are taken in the daytime is a problem for some patients. Daytime use of thyroid medication does not provide good FT3 levels when the adrenal glands are highly active during the latter part of the night. In many cases, inadequate cortisol levels are simply being caused by thyroid medication that fails to mimic healthy thyroid hormone levels. This <u>insight</u> explains why so many thyroid patients also have adrenal problems. This is a fundamental issue in the treatment of thyroid disease today! It explains why symptoms of partial adrenal insufficiency appear to be at epidemic levels amongst thyroid patients!

Stress, other health issues and ineffective thyroid treatment will also conspire to expose the potential for adrenal issues.

CT3M is closer to the healthy flow of thyroid hormone that would result in naturally high levels of free T3 in the night, thus supporting normal body functions like the production of cortisol by the adrenal glands.

CT3M is a good way of using NDT or T3 thyroid medication to achieve the natural peak level of FT3. Some thyroid patients never need to use CT3M, and are completely well dosing only during the daytime with thyroid medications like NDT and T3. However, it should be no surprise that some thyroid patients have partial adrenal insufficiency, because daytime only dosing may not reproduce healthy FT3 and cortisol levels.

CAN PEOPLE STOP CT3M ONCE THEIR CORTISOL IS NORMAL?

I have tried to stop using CT3M around a dozen times over the past fifteen years. Each time I have tried to do this my cortisol level has fallen, and I have become ill. I understand why this happens for me. I need to have high FT3 levels for my body to work right. If my FT3 is not high enough then I do not feel well. I also need to keep my FT3 high in the night when my adrenal glands begin to work.

Many thyroid patients using NDT or T3 medications find that they feel healthier with FT3 laboratory test results in the upper half or even upper quartile of the reference range, and in some cases above the top of the reference range. Many of these patients find that they also have partial adrenal insufficiency. This does not surprise me given the natural rhythm of thyroid hormones in healthy people (as described earlier). I think the simple act of introducing thyroid medications that create peak FT3 levels in the daytime may actually contribute partly to any partial adrenal insufficiency that may have already been there due to years of stress of one kind or another.

During thyroid treatment, if conditions change such that a thyroid patient no longer requires upper half or upper quartile FT3 levels to feel healthy, then they may at some point be able to stop using CT3M. For those patients with other health issues that have contributed to adrenal issues, then once these issues have been treated they may also be able to stop using CT3M. However, some individuals may continue to need CT3M indefinitely.

I believe that thyroid patients using CT3M may fall into one of three categories:

1.   Those that need to use CT3M to maintain a good level of FT3 when the adrenal glands begin to function. These people may need to keep using CT3M indefinitely. In some cases, other health issues may also need to be addressed before CT3M actually works properly.

2.   Those that use CT3M but have other health issues. When these health issues are resolved then these thyroid patients may be able to stop using CT3M.

3.   Those that use CT3M simply as a tool to wean adrenal steroids and glandulars. Once this is done they are able to stop using CT3M.

The above list is quite important and should be kept in mind. It is often not known which of these categories a thyroid patient may fall into when they start using CT3M. Only after much investigation and by observing actual results may this become clear.

CT3M DOES NOT WORK FOR EVERYONE

I began using CT3M about 15 years ago and I have had good health since that time. I have needed no adrenal support in the form of hydrocortisone or adrenal glandulars as a result. Yes - I've been using CT3M for well over a decade!

Since the release of *Recovering with T3*, many thyroid patients have used CT3M to improve their adrenal function and regain their health. Many have found that CT3M has been sufficient to allow them to wean adrenal glandulars, or steroids like hydrocortisone and florinef.

However, CT3M does not work for all. Health issues may need to be identified and resolved, and in some of these cases the health issues appear to be so chronic that even CT3M is not effective. CT3M is just one strategy that may be employed to improve adrenal health. Hopefully, over time, a more comprehensive health care approach will be developed that really does work for everyone.

IS CT3M AFFECTING THE ADRENALS OR THE HPA AXIS?

It is possible that CT3M has some effect on the hypothalamus and pituitary glands. However, there are a couple of arguments against this. If CT3M is really affecting the hypothalamic pituitary axis (HPA axis) then I'd expect higher TSH as well; this is something that is not seen. Also it's important to keep in mind that the pituitary is responsible for requesting the production of cortisol from the adrenal glands, which it does via the ACTH hormone (adrenocorticotropic hormone). The pituitary maintains the highest concentration of FT3 in the body, shown from dissection of different body tissues.[9] Even when FT3 is low in other tissues, including the adrenals, FT3 is still high in the pituitary. The reason for this is that the pituitary produces its own deiodinase enzymes and performs its own local FT4 to FT3 conversion. So, there is a high probability that for most adrenal fatigue patients, the pituitary is still doing a great job of making ACTH and thereby requesting cortisol be made by the adrenal glands.

Could CT3M be having an effect on hypothalamic and pituitary tissues? Yes, of course there could be some effect. However, I suspect that the effect of CT3M is directly on the adrenal glands.

More information may be found on CT3M on my website and in Appendix B.[10]

Chapter 3

Determining if CT3M is Relevant and Can Be Started

CT3M helps promote better adrenal production for thyroid patients who are experiencing partial adrenal insufficiency.

Before starting CT3M, the thyroid patient should take a twenty-four hour adrenal saliva test confirming there is partial adrenal insufficiency. For CT3M to be effective, the thyroid patient should have:

- Good iron levels, or be on iron supplementation. Some patients find that they need to improve iron levels before they can tolerate thyroid medication that contains T3. Others with low iron find that they can cope once they are taking iron supplements.
- Any existing blood sugar issues, such as pre-diabetes, diabetes or insulin resistance, in the process of being treated.
- Any sex hormone imbalances identified and ideally be in the process of correction, as these may disrupt thyroid hormone action.

In addition, CT3M must be used correctly, and patience is required to allow the adrenal glands time to work to their best ability.

CT3M IS UNLIKELY TO WORK WELL WITH ADDISON'S DISEASE

Addison's disease results in very low adrenal hormones from the adrenal cortex. Often cortisol, aldosterone and DHEA may be very low. Sometimes, only one of these may be low. Addison's disease is caused by destruction of the tissues of the adrenal glands. Frequently this is due to autoimmune attack, but tumours, physical injury or other diseases may also be the cause. The resulting low levels of adrenal hormones need to be replaced by drugs such as hydrocortisone and florinef, and this replacement will be for life.

The usual test for Addison's disease is run in a hospital or specialised clinic, and is known as an *ACTH stimulation test* or *Synacthen test*.

This test involves a series of blood samples. One blood sample is taken at the beginning of the test. Then a chemical is injected into the patient, which is either ACTH (the pituitary hormone that stimulates the production of cortisol), or a very similar chemical. Further blood samples are taken every half-an-hour thereafter. Typically three blood samples are taken following the injection of ACTH. The doctor interpreting the results uses the initial baseline level of cortisol, and the level of response to the injection, to assess the health of the adrenal glands and determine if there is a potentially serious adrenal issue.

Endocrinologists usually insist that the patient ceases the use of all adrenal hormones (e.g. HC, Florinef or adrenal glandulars), and even sex hormones (if they are being used), for a period of six weeks prior to the test. This is to avoid the results of the ACTH stimulation test being affected by these medications.

If the test is done properly and interpreted correctly, then it can be extremely useful in determining primary adrenal insufficiency due to destruction of the adrenal glands. However, the test does not rule out secondary adrenal insufficiency due to a hypothalamus or pituitary dysfunction.

An endocrinologist may occasionally decide to test for adrenal autoantibodies if Addison's disease is suspected. The most commonly tested of these are: adrenocortical autoantibodies (ACA), 21-hydroxy autoantibodies and the 21-OH autoantibodies. Two other autoantibodies that are associated with the adrenal glands, but are less frequently tested, are 17-alpha-hydroxylase and P450scc autoantibodies.

Addison's disease results in destruction of the tissues of the adrenal glands and this can take many years to progress. If this is due to attack by autoantibodies then it is important for the thyroid patient to do everything possible to calm the immune system down.

CT3M attempts to help the adrenal glands produce their hormones more effectively, but in the case where there is destruction of the adrenal tissues, CT3M may make little or no difference. Saying that, I have received reports from some thyroid patients who have an Addison's disease diagnosis, and are taking hydrocortisone, and they say that CT3M still helps them. This positive effect of CT3M may be due to the fact that they have sufficient remaining adrenal gland function and are not on a suppressive dosage of hydrocortisone. CT3M will not do any harm in the case of someone who has Addison's disease if the patient continues to take their adrenal hormone medication. In some cases where there is working adrenal tissue remaining, CT3M may help a little, but there is no guarantee of that.

CT3M IS UNLIKELY TO WORK WELL WITH HYPOPITUITARISM

In hypopituitarism, the pituitary gland does not send the correct level of one or more control signals that it is meant to send to organs like the adrenal glands. Hypopituitarism is sometimes referred to as secondary adrenal insufficiency.

Hypopituitarism can affect the thyroid gland, adrenals, and other endocrine glands (like the ovaries in women and the testes in men). It can affect one hormone only, or a range of hormones depending on the nature of the problem with the pituitary gland. Sometimes the hypothalamus can be part of the problem, as this important gland controls much of what the pituitary gland does.

If adrenal hormones or other hormones are sufficiently low then an endocrinologist or doctor may suspect hypopituitarism. They investigate this by measuring the levels of various hormones. In some cases, the results will clearly show hypopituitarism, whilst in others further testing may be required.

In the case of suspected hypopituitarism that may be affecting the adrenal glands, an endocrinologist may sometimes order a serum ACTH blood test. This is to examine the level of ACTH. An endocrinologist, who is unsure if primary or secondary adrenal insufficiency might be present, may ask for a serum ACTH test to be carried out just before an ACTH Stimulation test. However, even serum ACTH may not definitely prove that there is secondary adrenal insufficiency.

The most definitive test for secondary adrenal insufficiency (hypopituitarism) is an *insulin tolerance test* (ITT). This measures the adrenal glands' response to hypoglycaemia (low blood sugar/glucose levels).

Normally, the adrenals release extra cortisol when blood sugar falls below a certain level. This cortisol release raises blood sugar back up to a healthy level. However, weak adrenals are not as efficient at doing this. So this test aims to measure adrenal function by inducing a hypoglycaemic (low blood sugar) state.

The test itself involves taking a baseline cortisol level, and then injecting the patient with insulin so that they become hypoglycaemic. Cortisol blood samples are then taken every 15 minutes throughout the test and during the hypoglycaemia. Once hypoglycaemia has been achieved, the patient is injected with dextrose to bring the glucose levels up as quickly as possible. A nurse or doctor is present at all times throughout this test. They will take note of hypoglycaemic symptoms, as well as ensuring that the patient is rapidly given dextrose if they become unconscious. The ITT also measures growth hormone and insulin.

The ITT is considered the gold standard for diagnosing hypopituitarism and detecting hypothalamic-pituitary-adrenal axis problems. The test is extremely effective at detecting more subtle cases of adrenal insufficiency (and secondary adrenal insufficiency in particular). Therefore, it may be useful if partial adrenal insufficiency is suspected but the patient has not tested positive for Addison's disease. Many endocrinologists are reluctant to run an ITT, as it requires such close monitoring of the patient.

As with Addison's disease, CT3M will not harm a patient who has hypopituitarism. CT3M may have limited effect, though, if the hypopituitarism is so severe that there is little signal to the adrenal glands from the pituitary, or if the thyroid patient is on a level of adrenal medication that suppresses any remaining adrenal function.

PARTIAL ADRENAL INSUFFICIENCY

I developed CT3M to improve adrenal hormone production where partial adrenal insufficiency exists. Some thyroid patients refer to this as *adrenal fatigue,* or even *adrenal stress.* Doctors do not use the term adrenal fatigue and so I prefer to use the medical term *partial adrenal insufficiency.* Partial adrenal insufficiency can arise out of periods of sustained stress, or from incorrectly treated hypothyroidism. I developed CT3M many years ago specifically to treat my own partial adrenal insufficiency. It worked extremely well for me then, and it still does.

SYMPTOMS/CLUES SUGGESTING PARTIAL ADRENAL INSUFFICIENCY

The *Recovering with T3* book lists clues that suggest partial adrenal insufficiency may be present.[RWT3 1] Here is a summary of these clues.

Low cortisol clues: severe fatigue; low blood sugar (causing dizziness, a feeling of being unwell or hunger); aches/pains; dizziness; poor response to thyroid hormones; anxiety; irritability; panic; feeling cold; fluctuating body temperature; dark rings under the eyes; pale skin; skin appears thinner; digestive upsets or diarrhoea; allergies; flu-like symptoms; nausea; trembling or a jittery/hyper feeling; rapid heartbeat or pounding; difficulty sleeping; low blood pressure; low back pain (where the adrenal glands are located); worsening symptoms in the presence of stress of any kind, including minor infections.

Low aldosterone clues: low blood pressure (even lower if the blood pressure is taken immediately after the patient stands up (which is known as postural hypotension); craving for salty foods; thirst; dizziness when standing up; more frequent need to urinate or frequent urination during the night; excessive sweating; slightly higher body temperature than usual; high heart rate.

Fatigue and poor response to thyroid hormone treatment are often two of the big giveaways that adrenal issues exist:

1. Fatigue. Someone with hypothyroidism will usually feel better after a good night's sleep, usually becoming more tired/fatigued as the day goes on. If a thyroid patient feels exhausted upon waking and getting up out of bed in the morning then this is a good clue that partial adrenal insufficiency may exist.

2. Poor Response to Thyroid Hormone Treatment. If a thyroid patient fails to improve following an increase in their thyroid medication, then this can be a clue that adrenal issues exist. If the increased dosage produces a rapid heart rate in the presence of otherwise hypothyroid-like symptoms, then it is possible this is caused by adrenaline released due to a shortfall of cortisol. This type of response to thyroid treatment is fairly common in the presence of partial adrenal insufficiency, regardless of whether the treatment is NDT, T4/T3 or T3 replacement therapy.

If someone has enough evidence that partial adrenal insufficiency is present, it is essential to confirm this using a *twenty-four hour adrenal saliva test* (sometimes called an *adrenal stress test* by some laboratories).

LAB TESTING: TWENTY-FOUR HOUR ADRENAL SALIVA TEST, AND INTERPRETATION OF RESULTS

It is extremely important to have an adrenal saliva test before starting to use CT3M. This will show clearly whether there is partial adrenal insufficiency, and hence whether CT3M is genuinely applicable. If the thyroid patient's adrenal function is actually perfect, then the use of CT3M may cause cortisol levels to rise too high. Consequently, the twenty-four hour adrenal saliva test is a sensible precautionary lab test to do before commencing CT3M.

The twenty-four hour adrenal saliva test typically involves providing four separate saliva samples during the day, from morning to late evening, which are then sent off by mail to the specialist company. Results show the four distinct measures of free salivary cortisol at each point in the day. Typically, the private laboratory will provide a chart that illustrates how the patient's cortisol level appeared to fluctuate during the day, including any time periods when the cortisol was unusually high or low.

Blood testing of cortisol includes the measurement of cortisol bound to protein. This means that blood testing does not actually measure the biologically active cortisol. In addition to this, blood testing is usually only done once in the day, and therefore provides no profile of cortisol as it fluctuates over the patient's day.

We know from patient experience that adrenals that are under stress may produce very strange patterns of free cortisol. Sometimes a morning free cortisol result may look acceptable but the midday result can be extremely low. Sometimes the evening free cortisol can go high. For example, if a thyroid patient had very high cortisol in the evening (as determined by a twenty-four hour adrenal saliva test), then this insight would allow the use of supplements that might help to reduce this. This type of understanding is only possible through the use of a twenty-four hour adrenal saliva test.

Note, it is important for the thyroid patient not to be taking adrenal steroids of any kind, e.g. hydrocortisone or adrenal glandulars, for at least a week and ideally two-three weeks, before any adrenal saliva test. Doctors usually require patients to be off adrenal steroids for several weeks before ACTH Stimulation tests (Synacthen tests). Adrenal steroids should only be reduced and stopped under the supervision of the patient's own medical practitioner. Sometimes weaning adrenal steroids is not feasible, and so it is not possible to get an assessment of the function of the patient's adrenal health using an adrenal saliva test.

The experience of thyroid patients and doctors who regularly use adrenal saliva testing is that **healthy adrenal function** will typically exhibit the following pattern:

1. Early morning (approx. 8:00 am) result with free cortisol near the top of the reference range.
2. Late morning/lunchtime result with free cortisol in/near the upper quartile.
3. Late afternoon (approx. 5:00 pm) result with free cortisol around mid-range.
4. Late evening free cortisol near the bottom of the reference range.

CT3M has been used successfully with patterns of free cortisol that include low levels in the morning and/or noon. Sometimes CT3M has been attempted with some success with other patterns of free cortisol, but these should be discussed between the patient and their own doctor before attempting to use the CT3M option.

Clearly, judgment over the individual twenty-four hour adrenal saliva test results, and the presenting symptoms of the thyroid patient, is always required. However, it should be apparent that once partial adrenal insufficiency exists then one or more 'spikes' of high cortisol might also be present.

The twenty-four hour adrenal saliva test is very important and fortunately this is becoming more widely available these days. Although in some countries (including the UK), this often has to be done through a private test laboratory by sending the samples through the mail or by courier.

CT3M AND THYROID HORMONES MAY NOT WORK WELL IN THE PRESENCE OF LOW IRON LEVELS

This is covered in greater depth in *Recovering with T3*.[RWT3 2] There is also excellent information on this subject on the *Stop The Thyroid Madness* website, and within the *Stop The Thyroid Madness* book.[3, 4]

Iron is critical in order for thyroid hormone to work correctly. Therefore, iron levels need to be healthy for CT3M to have any chance of success. Consequently, a full iron panel should be done before starting CT3M. The most important iron tests to perform are:

*   Serum Iron.
*   Serum Ferritin.
*   Total Iron Binding Capacity.
*   Transferrin Saturation %.

These tests should be done as a set, which will then provide an extremely good picture of iron levels in the body and the level of iron supplementation required (if it is needed at all). **Note: All iron containing supplements must be stopped for at least a week (and ideally two-three weeks), before having iron tested, or the results will be influenced by supplementation.**

SERUM IRON

Typical laboratory reference ranges for serum iron are 65-176 ug/dL for men and 50-170 ug/dL for women. Serum iron is sometimes measured in umol/L; the reference range for women would then be 10-30 umol/L rather than 50-170 ug/dL. I have heard reports from other patients and Internet forums that suggest that thyroid patients feel better if their **serum iron is over 90 ug/dL (and ideally close to 100-110 ug/dL),** but still remaining within the laboratory reference range.

SERUM FERRITIN

Ferritin is a protein that stores iron within the tissues. It enables the steady release of iron, which our cells require. The serum ferritin blood test measures how much storage iron is available.

Typical laboratory reference ranges for serum ferritin are 22-320 ng/mL for men/post menopausal women and 10-290 ng/mL for pre menopausal women. However, many female thyroid patients report that their **serum ferritin needs to be at least in the 70 - 90 ng/mL range**, which is considerably higher than the lower reference range of most laboratories. Male thyroid patients do well with similar results, or even a little higher. If ferritin is 50 ng/mL or less, then this is too low, could be causing issues and may be suggesting that anaemia may ensue if iron levels fall lower. A level of 50 ng/mL is considered to be just getting by and iron supplementation should be considered.

However, with certain conditions serum ferritin may be misleading, for instance in the presence of inflammation (such as caused by Hashimoto's thyroiditis), infection or cancer. In the case of prolonged hypothyroidism, serum ferritin may be falsely elevated (or even sometimes low or normal), in the presence of both high and low iron levels. Inflammation caused by Hashimoto's thyroiditis, or caused by another health condition, can produce these falsely elevated ferritin levels. Consequently, in the first instance it is important to have the broad range of tests for iron as outlined here. In particular, the combination of serum iron, serum ferritin and transferrin saturation % may be more valuable in order to gain a more accurate appreciation of iron status. If low ferritin is present with high serum iron and high transferrin saturation %, then the patient's doctor must carefully assess whether this is simply a case of the ferritin level not yet being given adequate time to improve with iron supplementation, or whether some other process is at work.

TOTAL IRON BINDING CAPACITY (TIBC)

Total iron-binding capacity (TIBC) is most frequently used along with a serum iron test to evaluate people suspected of having either iron deficiency or iron overload. These two tests are used to calculate the transferrin saturation %, which is a more useful indicator of iron status than just iron or TIBC alone.

In iron deficiency, the serum iron level is often low, but the TIBC is increased. In states of excess iron, the serum iron level will be high, and the TIBC will be low, or normal. If TIBC is high, then there is likely to be a low amount of transferrin not carrying iron, i.e. the ability to carry additional iron is good. If TIBC is low, then the transferrin has limited capacity to bind further iron, i.e. the capacity of the blood to bind additional iron is poor.

If someone is identified as having a low iron level via one of the other tests, and a **low** level of TIBC is present, then the patient's doctor must take care when iron supplementation is started to avoid a build up of iron in the blood. In this case, iron supplementation must be far lower than is normally used for iron deficiency, and the building up of iron stores will take a lot longer to accomplish, e.g. less than 20 mg of elemental iron per day may be required initially until the TIBC becomes higher. In practice, thyroid patients have found that they appear to **handle iron supplementation reasonably well if their TIBC is at or above the lower quartile of the reference range**. The patient's doctor should be able to provide excellent advice on iron supplementation.

The typical reference range for TIBC is 240-450 ug/dL. Sometimes an alternative test called the UIBC is performed. This is the unsaturated iron binding capacity, and determines the reserve capacity of transferrin, i.e. the portion of transferrin that has not yet been saturated with iron. If serum iron and UIBC are known, then TIBC may be calculated as TIBC = UIBC + serum iron. The typical reference range for UIBC is 150-375 ug/dL.

TRANSFERRIN SATURATION %

Transferrin Saturation % = serum iron divided by TIBC x 100%. The transferrin saturation % tells a doctor how much of the free iron is being carried by transferrin. This is a far more useful indicator of iron status than just serum iron or TIBC alone.

Transferrin saturation % is sometimes referred to as the transferrin saturation index. For instance, a transferrin saturation % of 15% means that only 15% of the free iron is bound to transferrin. Typically the transferrin saturation % will be low if there is iron deficiency because serum iron will be low and TIBC will be high. The typical reference range for transferrin saturation % is 15-50% for men and 12-45% for women.

The feedback that I have received from experienced thyroid patients indicates that the transferrin saturation % should be maintained in the 25% - 45% range. However, recently I have read that some doctors in the USA have found that thyroid treatment proceeds more smoothly once the patient's **transferrin saturation % is in the 35% - 45% range, with serum iron ideally at least 90 ug/dL**. In this situation TIBC or UIBC may be low in their reference ranges, but still not below the lower end of the reference ranges. Transferrin saturation % should not exceed 45% though.

The above laboratory reference ranges are only typical and may vary depending on the laboratory performing the test.

If a thyroid patient does not have healthy iron levels then supplementing iron will be needed in order to enable CT3M to work correctly. Testing iron levels properly is essential before starting CT3M, as thyroid hormone action will be undermined if iron levels are low. This will lead to a poor response to CT3M, wasted time and frustration for the thyroid patient.

Once iron has been tested properly and found to be low then supplementation of iron should be started. Once supplementation is in place then iron may be re-tested in a few months, taking care to stop the iron supplementation for a week, and ideally 2-3 weeks, prior to the iron test.

Unfortunately, the experience of many thyroid patients is that they do not get the complete set of iron tests, and that a laboratory test result that barely creeps into the low end of a reference range is taken as being an acceptable level of iron! Sometimes, a thyroid patient has to become very assertive in order to get the correct testing and supplementation regime that they really need.

CT3M may be started even if iron is low, as long as the supplementation with iron has begun. Care should be taken not to raise the circadian dose too quickly, or too high.

OTHER LAB TESTS TO DO BEFORE STARTING CT3M

There are many laboratory tests available these days. Due to their own particular medical condition(s), each patient may have specific tests that are clearly relevant to themselves. However, it is often advisable for the thyroid patient to test the following before starting CT3M:

- B12.[RWT3 5]
- Folate. Folic acid is necessary for the body to utilise vitamin B12.[RWT3 5]
- Vitamin D. The 25-hydroxy vitamin D test provides insight into vitamin D levels in the body. Low vitamin D can hamper thyroid hormone action.[RWT3 5]

All of the above may be supplemented if they are found to be low.

CT3M MAY NOT WORK WELL IF THERE ARE BLOOD SUGAR ISSUES

The most important point to mention here is that **good blood sugar control is essential** to the action of all thyroid hormones. This is not specific to CT3M at all. A good flow of glucose from the bloodstream into the cells enables the cells to produce a substance called adenosine triphosphate (ATP). ATP is what one thyroid patient described to me as the, 'spark of life' in our cells. It is the raw form of chemical energy that our cells use. Without a good level of ATP, thyroid hormone just won't work correctly.

Consequently, the correct management of blood sugar from digested food to the bloodstream, and through healthy insulin and cortisol action, is essential for thyroid hormones to work. This is not specific to CT3M, but if blood sugar issues exist then they will undermine CT3M and may prevent the desired improvement in adrenal health.

If a blood sugar issue is suspected, then it should be tested thoroughly. If there is a problem, a treatment regime should be put in place before starting CT3M. I will say far more about blood sugar later in Chapter 7.

SEX HORMONES

An imbalance of one or more sex hormones can adversely affect the action of thyroid hormone and the adrenal glands. Proper testing of sex hormones is the way to ensure that any imbalances are detected.[RWT3 6] With the support of a competent doctor, any imbalance may be corrected. This correction may often be achieved through the use of bio-identical hormone replacement.

Chapter 4

CT3M Whilst Taking Adrenal Hormones

This chapter is mainly in place for those thyroid patients who do not have Addison's disease or hypopituitarism, and for one reason or another are taking adrenal steroids to support adrenal function (and not for medical conditions that require these).

Throughout *The CT3M Handbook*, I try to avoid the use of the term *adrenal fatigue*. The reason for this is that doctors and endocrinologists do not understand it, or accept it as a medical condition. I prefer to use *partial adrenal insufficiency*, it is less ambiguous, is understood, and is also accepted by the medical profession. **However, the reader should be aware that I consider the terms *partial adrenal insufficiency* and *adrenal fatigue* to refer to the same condition.**

If a thyroid patient has been found to have low cortisol levels (as revealed by a twenty-four hour adrenal saliva test), it is always advisable to have a Synacthen test. The Synacthen test, which is also known as an ACTH stimulation test, rules out Addison's disease. Low cortisol levels may also be caused by hypopituitarism, which results in too low an ACTH signal being sent to the adrenal glands. This in turn causes too little cortisol and other adrenal hormones to be produced. Hypopituitarism is quite rare, but if suspected by a patient's doctor then it may be tested via an Insulin Tolerance Test.

If Addison's disease and hypopituitarism are unlikely, or have been excluded by laboratory test, then CT3M should be far more likely to be helpful.

I do know of some thyroid patients who have been diagnosed with either Addison's disease or hypopituitarism, who have combined their steroid treatment with CT3M. They have found that there was some benefit to this, but there is no guarantee that this would work for the majority of thyroid patients. However, CT3M should not be harmful even if a patient had Addison's disease or hypopituitarism, as long as the existing medication to treat these conditions was not withdrawn. More on this may be found in Chapters 12 and 22.

Some thyroid patients may also require prescribed adrenal steroids due to other diagnosed medical conditions. Some inflammatory diseases require the use of adrenal steroids for life.

Patients who are considering CT3M need to be aware that the use of adrenal steroids or adrenal glandulars may be suppressing their adrenal glands. They may prevent CT3M from having any effect at all. Some of these thyroid patients may have been encouraged by reading Internet articles, or by fellow patients, to use steroids like hydrocortisone in order to 'rest' their adrenal glands and give them some time to 'recover'. Personally, I don't believe that most thyroid patients need to do this. Using CT3M, thyroid patients often recover from supposedly 'tired' adrenal glands without any need to 'rest' them. **CT3M works especially well if someone actually uses it before ever having gone on adrenal steroids and as soon as adrenal issues are recognised.**

The idea behind using adrenal steroids (like hydrocortisone) or adrenal glandular products for partial adrenal insufficiency (not proper Addison's disease or hypopituitarism) is to replace any adrenal steroid deficit that may be present. There is an inherent problem with this approach. When adrenal steroids or adrenal glandulars are taken, there is a feedback mechanism that is affected. The pituitary gland 'sees' more adrenal steroids in the bloodstream and 'says' to the adrenals, "OK! I don't need to ask for as much cortisol now." The consequence is even less demand for cortisol and other steroids from the adrenals. What does that do? What does any organ do if it isn't used as much? It can become even more weak and sluggish.

In the case of the adrenals, the thyroid patient can become very dependent on adrenal steroids and may never be able to stop using them. Far from being a temporary solution to 'rest tired adrenal glands', the thyroid patient may become dependent on the use of adrenal steroids and adrenal glandular products for the long-term. For long-term users of adrenal steroids or adrenal glandulars, CT3M may not work as well as it does for other thyroid patients experiencing some partial adrenal insufficiency. There is also the concern that after long term use of adrenal steroids, the adrenal glands themselves may exhibit atrophy as a result of the extended period of less than natural action.

I've spoken to hundreds of thyroid patients who have had adrenal problems. Many of these have at one time or another been on adrenal steroids (hydrocortisone or florinef), or adrenal glandulars. Very few of these thyroid patients have ever failed a Synacthen test. Their adrenals have responded (when demanded to) with ACTH! There has been no fundamental adrenal damage and yet for one reason or another many have taken adrenal steroids or glandulars, often out of desperation.

I am not against adrenal steroid or adrenal glandular use for those thyroid patients that need them, but so many people have been encouraged to use these when they don't actually have adrenal damage or hypopituitarism - this does not seem a good idea to me.

As explained in Chapter 2, CT3M attempts to mimic nature and raise FT3 levels during the night. CT3M is sometimes the only correction that is needed for partial adrenal insufficiency. However, CT3M does not always work. For some thyroid patients there are other health problems that may need addressing before the partial adrenal insufficiency responds to CT3M. These issues are covered in more detail in Chapter 8. In some cases the underlying health issue may be hard to discover, or may never be discovered, and CT3M may not resolve the patient's issues.

In general, the use of adrenal steroids and CT3M together is not a very sensible option. This is because steroids in the form of synthetic medication like hydrocortisone, or in the form of adrenal glandulars, have a suppressive effect on normal adrenal gland function. Having said that, I do know of a few thyroid patients who cannot function well without the use of adrenal steroids, and who are able to use CT3M. Some of these have an Addison's disease diagnosis but still have some adrenal function remaining. These patients appear to obtain some benefit from the use of CT3M combined with their adrenal steroids or adrenal glandular products, but this is not a typical approach with CT3M.

Chapter 5

Thyroid Medications for CT3M

The two thyroid medications that may successfully be used for CT3M are standard T3 (also known as pure T3) and natural desiccated thyroid (NDT). Both of these medications work well for the circadian dose (the early morning dose taken during the last four hours of sleep). The choice between the two can depend on whether the patient has any problems with the processing or conversion of T4 to T3, or with reverse T3.

The choices and combinations for the circadian and daytime doses that I'm aware are used by thyroid patients are:
- A pure T3 circadian dose, and daytime doses of either T3 or NDT.
- NDT for both the circadian dose and daytime doses.
- T3 for the circadian dose, and T4 for the daytime dose.
- A circadian dose only of either T3 or NDT, with no daytime dose of thyroid medication. These patients tend only to have weak adrenals, and not thyroid issues.
- A combination of NDT and T3 taken together as a circadian dose, i.e. a single dose, but with a combination of different medication types. This seems a little over-complicated, but if it works well then that is fine. This approach may be used for the daytime doses; alternatively either pure T3 or pure NDT doses may be used.

Very often the only way to establish the optimal combination of thyroid medication is to find out through practical experience. The typical order in which various combinations of thyroid medication are tried is:
1. NDT for all thyroid medication - both the circadian dose and daytime doses.
2. T3 for the circadian dose; NDT for daytime doses.
3. T3 for all thyroid medication - both the circadian dose and daytime doses.

In my own experience I have found that options 2 and 3 appear to be most effective. For people with chronic health issues, then option 3 is often more effective. Most of the complete health recoveries that I have witnessed with thyroid patients using CT3M have been when they were using T3 only for both the circadian and daytime doses (option 3). However, I have seen some with the other two options also.

SLOW RELEASE T3 AND SUB-LINGUAL ABSORPTION OF T3/NDT ARE A NO-NO

In *Recovering with T3,* I describe the arrival of a dose of T3 akin to a wave that has to reach the interior of the cells.[RWT3 1] Slow release T3 (also known as sustained release T3) is incapable of being fine-tuned to deliver an ideal sized 'wave' of T3. This means that slow release T3 is fundamentally a poor tool for the treatment of 'impaired cellular response to thyroid hormone'. If too low a dose of slow release T3 is used, then the cells never receive enough T3 to work correctly. If a high enough dose of slow release T3 is used, then frequently there are times when it is too high and tissue over-stimulation can occur.

Attempts to use sub-lingual absorption of T3 or NDT for the circadian dose may also have serious problems. Sub-lingual absorption may result in a slow drip feed of T3 into the cells, rather than the relatively fast arrival of a properly swallowed dose of pure T3 or NDT. This is especially true during the night when our mouths produce less saliva and may remain drier.

CT3M needs all the T3 in the circadian dose to arrive quickly at the correctly determined time in order to support the adrenal glands. Consequently, slow release thyroid medications and sub-lingual absorption are far less effective. It is better to swallow the circadian dose in one go and wash it down with a little water.

THYROID MEDICATION ON THE DAY OF LAB TESTING

One question that frequently comes up is whether a thyroid patient should take their circadian dose on the morning prior to a laboratory test. The answer to this question really depends on the laboratory test that is being run.

For an adrenal saliva test, or cortisol blood test, then it is generally better to see what the patient's cortisol levels are like with CT3M in place. Hence the circadian dose should remain in place and the thyroid patient should take their normal doses of T3 or NDT at the usual times that they take them.

For other forms of adrenal testing, such as a Synacthen test, then the patient's endocrinologist may wish to make the decision to either continue the normal medication dosing or not. This will depend on whether they wish to see the worst case response of the adrenal glands (no CT3M), or best case response (with CT3M).

Thyroid hormone blood tests (TSH, FT4, FT3 or reverse T3) are frequently done during the morning. The use of a circadian dose of either T3 or NDT will often cause FT3 to rise sharply to the top of the reference range, or even beyond it by the time of the blood draw. This rapid rise in FT3 can also cause TSH to be suppressed to a very low level (perhaps between 1.0 and 0) for some few hours after the circadian dose. Consequently, the choice of whether to take a circadian dose on the morning of the laboratory test may require some judgement depending on what is trying to be discovered during the testing.

Many thyroid patients and their doctors do not wish to measure peak FT3 levels, preferring to see a more average level of FT3 and TSH. As a result they often decide to skip the circadian dose on the morning of the blood draw. Sometimes the last T3-containing medication is only taken prior to 6 pm on the day before the thyroid hormone blood test, if FT3 and TSH are being measured.

For the testing of thyroid autoantibodies and of FT4, there should be no need to suspend the use of the circadian dose on the morning of the test.

Chapter 6

Essential Supplements

In *Recovering with T3,* I discuss the importance of addressing nutrient deficiencies and the preparatory steps for using T3.[RWT3 1] These preparatory steps are also useful before starting CT3M (with T3 or NDT). I do not intend to repeat the same level or degree of detail here, as *The CT3M Handbook* is intended to be used alongside *Recovering with T3,* and not to replace it.

I will assume that the important nutrient tests discussed in Chapter 3 of this book have been completed, and that any necessary supplementation of nutrients like iron or B12 has been carried out under the supervision of the patient's doctor.

This short chapter is therefore just a brief reminder that there are many important vitamins and minerals that are critical to thyroid hormone action. If these vitamins and minerals are already in the patient's diet in healthy quantities then this is excellent. If they are not then the patient should consider supplementing them. Patients have multiple ways of handling this, including working with their doctor or a qualified nutritionist.

In *Recovering with T3,* I discuss the supplements that I have personally found to be important in order to reduce or eliminate problems:

- Strong B complex. High levels of all the main B vitamins, e.g. 50 mg B1, B2, B3, B5 and B6. These B vitamins are **crucial** for the adrenal and thyroid pathways to function correctly and they are critical to energy production.
- Vitamin B12. The level depends on the result of a B12 test. If B12 is deficient, then the patient's doctor should establish a treatment. If the B12 test is normal, then some low level of B12 supplementation e.g. 500 micrograms daily, may still make sense to ensure it cannot develop into a problem during thyroid treatment. The B12 and folate tests (folic acid or B9) sometimes do not reflect actual cellular levels of these B vitamins - more on this later in Chapter 8.
- Vitamin C. Taken 4 to 6 times per day in divided doses of 500 milligrams each.
- Vitamin D3. How much depends on the result of a vitamin D test. If the vitamin D levels are low, then the patient's doctor will advise treatment. I have successfully used vitamin D3 supplementation of 2500 IUs of vitamin D3 during the months when there is less natural sunlight (October to March in the UK), and I stop taking vitamin D3

in the months when there is more natural sunlight available (April to September in the UK).

- A good quality multi-mineral with a wide range of macro and trace minerals.
- Magnesium. Supplementation of magnesium at 400-1000 milligrams per day. I have found that chelated magnesium is easier on the digestive system, and I now use 200 milligrams of chelated magnesium twice a day (as well as the small amount in my multi-mineral). From the non-chelated products, magnesium citrate is thought to be well absorbed.
- Any other specific nutrients that have been found to be deficient from the nutrient testing, e.g. folic acid if the folate test indicated it was low or iron.

Readers should consult their own personal physician to ensure that any supplements they are considering taking are safe. Furthermore, that they are being taken in safe quantities, and will have no adverse interactions with other medications or conditions that they may have.

Thyroid patients should also be aware that some doctors believe that a nutrient may be at a healthy level if a laboratory test result is near the bottom of the reference range. This can leave the patient with a very low level of an important vitamin or mineral, and with the patient's doctor thinking that the patient is OK. This is a cautionary note for thyroid patients to do their own research and not simply accept everything that they are told. Good examples of this are when iron, B12 or vitamin D results are low, but still within the reference range. In these cases, there should be some supplementation to raise the vitamin or mineral to a healthy level in the upper half of the reference range. However, many thyroid patients may be told they do not require supplementation simply because the lab test result crept into the bottom of the reference range!

The above approach is designed to ensure that the thyroid and adrenal metabolic pathways are well resourced with the important nutrients in order to minimise problems during the application of CT3M. It may seem a step that is worth skipping, but this can cost a significant amount of time later if problems result that turn out to be due to a nutrient deficiency.

Chapter 7

Blood Sugar, Insulin and Cortisol

I wrote about this topic in the *Recovering with T3* book.[RWT3 1] However, it is clear from listening to many thyroid patients since *Recovering with T3* was published, that blood sugar balance is a problem that can affect thyroid hormone treatment far more profoundly than patients and some doctors actually realise.

DIGESTION AND DIGESTIVE SYSTEM HEALTH

When someone begins to eat, food is initially broken into pieces in the mouth and saliva begins the process of digestion. In the stomach, the acid and digestive juices begin to churn the food into a creamy mixture known as *chyme*. The enzyme pepsin is also released in the stomach and this breaks down protein. Consequently, adequate stomach acid and pepsin are important in the digestion process. Food can stay in the stomach for several minutes or several hours.

After the partly digested food in the chyme is released from the stomach it enters the small intestine. The digestion and absorption of fats, proteins and carbohydrates occurs within the small intestine. The gallbladder delivers bile salts that help to make fats easier to absorb. The pancreas produces bicarbonate, which neutralises the acidic chyme from the stomach: it also delivers digestive enzymes into the small intestine. The wall of the small intestine contains cells that produce enzymes that further digest the food and neutralise the acid. The inner surface of the small intestine contains hair-like structures called villi, which greatly increase the surface area available for absorption. Blood vessels receive the nutrition from the digested food via the villi, and then the nutrients are transported through the bloodstream to the liver. Various 'friendly' bacteria and other 'friendly' microorganisms live in the small intestine. Friendly bacteria are vital for the immune system: they protect against 'unfriendly' microorganisms that can cause disease, and they take part in the digestion and the absorption of food.

The unabsorbed residue of this process finally reaches the end of the small intestine and enters the large intestine. The large intestine contains hundreds of different species of bacteria that break down and utilise the undigested residues from our food, mostly dietary fibres. As the watery contents move along the large intestine the water content is absorbed. The residue stored as faeces in the rectum is eventually excreted.

For thyroid patients it is important to remember that thyroid hormone itself is absorbed in the small intestine. Vitamins and minerals that need to be absorbed from food or supplements also have to be absorbed in the small intestine. **Glucose must rise in the bloodstream as a result of eating and digesting food for thyroid hormones to work correctly.** All parts of the digestive system need to be working well for this rise in blood sugar to occur. This includes adequate stomach acid and pepsin levels, as well as good intestinal health. Good intestinal health requires adequate levels of digestive enzymes and the right balance of friendly microorganisms; these aid digestion and provide protection from unfriendly microorganisms. The friendly bacteria and other microorganisms in the gut are critical to the maintenance of gut integrity. In addition to this, there must be a good supply of nutrients, proteins, carbohydrates and fats in the diet for the body to function well. Consequently, a well balanced diet that provides adequate levels of protein, carbohydrates and fat is also important.

INTRODUCING ATP

Cells need to be able to create a source of chemical energy called adenosine triphosphate (ATP). When thyroid hormone attaches to the receptors within our cell nuclei and attempts to transcribe the genes to regulate cell function, there has to be enough ATP present for the nucleus and other entities to use. If insufficient glucose enters the cells, the mitochondria within our cells cannot make enough ATP. If there is not enough ATP, then thyroid hormone will not be able to create the necessary response.

The above means that if a thyroid patient is not producing enough ATP, an increase in the level of thyroid medication they are taking may not produce any noticeable effect and the patient may remain with hypothyroid symptoms. This could be the case even if the patient's thyroid blood test results appeared completely healthy!

LOOKING AT INSULIN, CORTISOL, BLOOD SUGAR AND ATP

This is a simplified description of one of the many complex systems in the human body. However, I will discuss enough so that the importance of blood sugar management, good diet, digestive system health, good production/response to insulin, adequate cortisol and mitochondrial health will become apparent.

As a result of adequate food intake and good digestion, blood sugar levels will rise. The pancreas releases insulin as a result of rising glucose (blood sugar). Insulin causes some of this blood sugar to be stored in the body for later use (mostly as glycogen, a molecule that contains glucose). **Insulin also interacts with the membrane around each cell in our body to allow some glucose to enter the cell.** If the insulin is too low, or does not interact correctly with the walls of our cells, then insufficient glucose will enter our cells.

Each cell of our body contains an entity called a mitochondrion. Collectively, the mitochondria are responsible for producing the energy that each cell needs in order to perform its specific functions (often this is the production of specific types of proteins e.g. muscle cells produce proteins that are specific to them as opposed to brain cells). The chemical energy that the mitochondria produce is called adenosine triphosphate (ATP).

The mitochondria use various co-factors in the production of ATP. These co-factors include L-carnitine, coenzyme Q-10, NADH, B complex vitamins, lipoic acid, magnesium and various other nutrients. **In addition to these co-factors, the mitochondria require a good supply of glucose.** If glucose in the blood does not continue to flow into the cells, then the production of ATP may reduce.

Hours after a meal, blood sugar levels will decline. This may be a frequent occurrence if the digestive system is not healthy, or if someone is on a diet that is not delivering enough blood sugar after meals. **When blood sugar levels fall, then the adrenals are asked to make more cortisol.** One of the main functions of cortisol is a process, called glucogenesis (making glucose).

Cortisol helps to release stored glucose from glycogen, and via this process blood glucose is maintained at a high enough level that some glucose continues to be made available to our cells. Insulin is released as discussed above, and the interaction of insulin with our cell membranes should allow this glucose to flow into our cells.

Thus a splendid dance of good diet, healthy digestive system activity, glucose in the blood, cortisol, insulin and mitochondrial function ensure cellular energy in the form of ATP is always available to our cells.

IMPORTANCE TO THYROID HORMONE

Thyroid hormone is used within our cells in two important ways:

1. It binds to receptors in the mitochondria, enabling the mitochondria to make enough ATP.
2. It binds to receptors in the cell nuclei, enabling the cell to perform its role.

It is through binding to the receptors in the cell nuclei and in the mitochondria that thyroid hormone regulates our metabolic rate. If there is too little thyroid hormone action within our cells, then we will develop symptoms of hypothyroidism. **This intra-cellular action of thyroid hormones is what counts - not circulating blood levels of thyroid hormone.**

The most biologically active thyroid hormone is T3, which is around ten times more metabolically potent than T4. Research studies have measured the potency of T3 in terms of its effect on the regulation of cell function. Some people, even doctors, believe that T3 is only four to five times the potency of T4, but this is not accurate. When a healthy thyroid gland is producing thyroid hormone, the thyroid will make four to five times the volume of T4 relative to its T3 production. This should not be confused with the potency of T3, compared with T4.

In addition to the above, T3 also binds more easily to the receptors in the cells than T4, so there is an argument that T3 is even more potent than this ten-times-T4 figure.

T4, T3 and reverse T3 (rT3) all try to bind to the thyroid receptors within the cells. If there is some imbalance within the cells that results in too little active T3 (relative to the metabolism slowing effect of any rT3), the symptoms of hypothyroidism can result.

I also harbour a deep suspicion, which is based on my experience and the experience of hundreds of other thyroid patients who have resorted to using T3 replacement therapy. This suspicion is that too much T4 hormone can have a negative effect on cell metabolism for some thyroid patients. I believe that some thyroid patients need as little interference by T4 and rT3 hormones within the cells as possible, in order that the potent T3 hormone can have an adequate effect. This is only my personal opinion. It would require a great deal of laboratory research to be carried out in order to prove it operates this way for some thyroid patients.

There is no laboratory test that exists at the present time to measure the precise activity levels of thyroid hormones either inside the cells, or at the cell nuclei and mitochondria. Thyroid blood tests show circulating levels of thyroid hormone only, and although they can often be used to manage thyroid treatment, the results of these laboratory tests can be unrepresentative of actual thyroid hormone activity inside our cells. For more information on this, please read the *Recovering with T3* book.

Our cells will not respond correctly to thyroid hormone if there is not enough ATP. We can have perfectly adequate thyroid medication of the right type for us, but if there is not enough ATP then we will remain with symptoms associated with hypothyroidism.

ATP may be low if there are problems with the mitochondria themselves. This is rare and will not be discussed further in this chapter. Many other things can go wrong, and these issues may affect the action of thyroid hormone generally (not just CT3M). If pre-diabetes (beginning of issues with low insulin), diabetes, insulin resistance (insulin not correctly affecting the cell membranes), digestive system issues, or low cortisol exist and are not treated, then insufficient ATP is the result and thyroid hormone will not work properly.

LOW ATP AND ADRENALINE

If ATP becomes too low within the cells, the body attempts to correct this by creating more glucose through the production of adrenaline. Hence situations of low cortisol, insulin deficiency (pre-diabetes or diabetes that is untreated), or untreated insulin resistance (IR) can result in adrenaline release in an attempt by the body to raise blood sugar. This adrenaline release may cause the all too familiar symptoms of raised heart rate, raised blood pressure, excess nervous energy and even facial flushing.

Many thyroid patients have experienced these symptoms, and more often than not they may have assumed it is due to too much thyroid hormone, or a lack of tolerance to their thyroid medication. However, these symptoms can be the result of adrenaline release due to low glucose within the cells and a consequent low ATP production. Problems with the digestive system and very low food intake can cause the same problems.

LABORATORY TESTING CAN BE HELPFUL

If excess adrenaline is suspected, or thyroid hormone response is not what is expected after most of the common problems have been excluded, then it may be worth looking more closely at blood sugar control. A glucose tolerance test (GTT) should be able to provide valuable information on this. A GTT measures blood glucose levels several times over a period of hours.

The patient has to fast beforehand and so the GTT is normally carried out first thing in the morning. Blood is drawn, a measured amount of glucose is given, and the rise and fall of blood sugar is recorded after fixed intervals of time. If insulin is also measured alongside the glucose readings, then this can provide particularly insightful data. However, this is something that a patient would have to ask their doctor to do, as usually glucose only is measured in a GTT. A comprehensive GTT can detect issues such as insulin resistance and pre-diabetes.

SHORT DISCUSSION ON INSULIN RESISTANCE

There are probably several causes of insulin resistance, and there is thought to be a strong genetic factor (an inherited component). Some medications can also lead to insulin resistance. In addition, insulin resistance is often seen in the following conditions:
* Metabolic syndrome.
* Obesity.
* Pregnancy.
* Infection or severe illness.
* Stress.
* During steroid use (perhaps from high cortisol and/or the early stage of adrenal problems).

It is stress and steroid use that particularly come to my mind when thinking about thyroid patients and insulin resistance. I am aware of a large number of thyroid patients who have been diagnosed with insulin resistance. I believe that this may be linked to past stress and periods of elevated cortisol. In the evolution of adrenal problems due to stress, it is very common for there to be periods of time during which the individual has higher than normal cortisol. I suspect this is at least one connection to the start of insulin resistance for some thyroid patients. Consequently, I believe that adrenal issues can cause insulin resistance, and insulin resistance can cause adrenal issues. If partial adrenal insufficiency begins to occur, then the body may become dependent on adrenaline to raise blood glucose. This is thought by some to make insulin resistance more likely because adrenaline spikes raise blood sugar rapidly. This rapid and potentially high rise of blood sugar may create more of a demand for insulin, and thus the environment for insulin resistance may be created.

Fortunately, there are various approaches to dealing with insulin resistance, including drugs like Metformin. This can help to reduce the insulin levels in the body and make any insulin we produce work more efficiently. Some thyroid patients believe that alpha lipoic acid may also offer some value.

I have seen some thyroid patients struggling to achieve a proper response to thyroid hormone (including CT3M), who have eventually been diagnosed with insulin resistance. In many cases the correct diagnosis and treatment (often with drugs like Metformin) can enable far more effective thyroid hormone action, including a more effective response to CT3M.

CAUTION ON MANAGING BLOOD SUGAR WITH LOW CARB DIETS

If a thyroid patient has issues with elevated blood sugar, then they may often be told that this might develop into diabetes or into insulin resistance. I frequently come across thyroid patients who have been encouraged by their doctors (or others) to use a low carbohydrate diet. Often this type of diet may have been a personal choice of the thyroid patient, perhaps due to weight gain. For a thyroid patient who may not be responding well to thyroid hormone treatment, this chapter should have already provided enough information to point out the potential pitfall in the use of a low carbohydrate diet. However, I will spell this out.

If the symptoms of hypothyroidism remain regardless of the thyroid medication that the patient is using, then the last thing they should be doing is further limiting the potential for ATP production. A low carbohydrate diet will be effective at keeping blood sugar lower - there is no doubt of this. It may be so effective that blood sugar does not rise as it is supposed to after a meal. This in turn can limit the normal process of insulin release and the flow of glucose into the cells to the mitochondria. The resulting lower production of ATP will potentially stifle the action of thyroid hormone.

Some thyroid patients remain healthy on a low carbohydrate diet because their metabolism has margin to cope. In fact, some patients do better on high protein, good quality fat and low carb diets, perhaps due to poor blood sugar metabolism. However, some are not; a low carbohydrate diet or a diet that is providing too little nutrition will simply keep them in a state where they continue to experience symptoms of hypothyroidism.

For those patients with blood sugar balance issues who remain with hypothyroid symptoms, then it may be far more effective to determine the exact cause of the blood sugar imbalance and then treat it. The goal should not simply be to keep a thyroid patient's blood sugar low, but to actually have the patient feeling well.

GTT AND ITT LABORATORY TESTS

For completeness, I will briefly discuss two laboratory tests that are sometimes confused with each other.

A glucose tolerance test (GTT) involves fasting and then a measured amount of glucose is given. Insulin should rise, causing blood glucose levels to fall over a few hours. If glucose is measured every hour for 2 - 6 hours, then the normal pattern of rising and falling glucose levels should be seen. If blood sugar falls too slowly, then pre-diabetes, diabetes or insulin resistance may be a diagnosis. If the doctor organising the test can be persuaded to also measure insulin during this process, then the diagnosis can be even more confident. A GTT won't tell you about the health of the mitochondria inside the cells that are responsible for making ATP, but it will highlight any issues with pre-diabetes or insulin resistance.

An insulin tolerance test (ITT) is a test for hypopituitarism. It involves giving the patient an injection of insulin, which rapidly lowers blood glucose levels. This rapid reduction of blood glucose creates a demand for the pituitary to respond with ACTH. ACTH (adrenocorticotropic hormone) is the hormone signal from the pituitary gland that asks the adrenal glands to manufacture and release more cortisol. The adrenal glands then have to respond to the ACTH request. An ITT is the gold standard test for hypopituitarism. An ITT can also identify partial adrenal insufficiency. It is a difficult test to do, and the patient has to be watched carefully because it can result in coma. Most doctors don't want to do this because of the risks, but if the patient is taken care of properly, then this is an excellent test when hypopituitarism or partial adrenal insufficiency needs to be investigated. It is an entirely different laboratory test to a GTT.

A GTT is something that may be highly useful if someone is not responding well to thyroid treatment, and blood sugar issues are a possibility. An ITT should only be done if hypopituitarism, or partial adrenal insufficiency, is suspected that other cortisol tests have not been able to confirm.

Chapter 8

20 Situations or Conditions That Can Undermine CT3M

This chapter can be read as part of the introductory information in this section of *The CT3M Handbook*, or alternatively it may be skipped by the reader (or skim read) and read later if progress has not been made with CT3M.

There are many things that can interfere with thyroid hormone action within the human body. CT3M is the application of thyroid hormone during the period of time when the adrenal glands are working extremely hard to produce the early morning high volume of cortisol. Consequently, if problems exist that might interfere with thyroid hormone action, then these are just as likely to interfere with CT3M. Some conditions that affect the adrenal glands directly will also have the potential to prevent CT3M from helping.

The situations or medical conditions that are now known or suspected to interfere with the effectiveness of CT3M are numerous, and include:

- Inadequate thyroid hormone treatment during the daytime.
- Highly irregular sleeping / waking pattern.
- Low iron.
- Methylation defects.
- Vitamin B Complex, B12, or folate deficiency.
- Other nutrient deficiencies.
- Blood sugar metabolism issues.
- Mercury / heavy metal toxicity.
- Fluoride toxicity.
- Sex hormone imbalances.
- Undiagnosed hypopituitarism or HPA axis problems.
- Undiagnosed Addison's disease.
- Use of anti-depressants.
- Lowered cortisol due to the unhelpful side effect of some nutrients.
- Digestive system conditions or gut integrity issues.
- Chronic inflammation issues.
- Low levels of related adrenal hormones.
- Mitochondrial disease or issues.
- Immune system hyper-activity.

- Some bacterial or viral infections.

... I fully expect that others will be discovered.

Some thyroid patients respond well to CT3M and see immediate improvement in their health. Other thyroid patients experience little or no improvement in their health until one or more other health conditions are identified and addressed. Unfortunately, for those individuals who have been ill for a long time, some of whom may have been using adrenal steroids for many years, more than one chronic condition may be present. Adrenal steroid use (when they are not required) may damage gut health, have an impact on the immune system and suppress adrenal gland function. Consequently, it is important to see CT3M as one strategy amongst many to deal with partial adrenal insufficiency and to help the proper function of thyroid hormone.

CT3M will not work in all cases of partial adrenal insufficiency. However, CT3M is relatively easy to attempt. Since CT3M does help many thyroid patients, it is a good option to have in the toolkit for dealing with partial adrenal insufficiency.

APPROACH TO DISCUSSING EACH SITUATION OR CONDITION

In Chapter 1, I stated that *The CT3M Handbook* is intended to be a practical book, with far fewer pages than *Recovering with T3*. I have also written each chapter to be as short as possible so that the book can be easily digestible in bite-size chunks. In order to do this, I have made the decision to almost completely avoid the provision of supporting evidence and medical references.

This chapter is a good example of a chapter where a great deal could be written on each situation or condition. Some conditions or topics are so large that they could have their own books written on them! I have written as little on each of these situations or conditions as I could do in order to meet my goals. The consequence of this is that further research will need to be done by any reader if they suspect that one or more of these health issues might apply to them. I realise that this will frustrate some people who will want more information, but I believe it is the right choice. My intention is to raise awareness of these situations and conditions, such that they can be looked into further by the patient if it seems relevant.

The CT3M Handbook is just that - it is a focused book on CT3M. It is not a comprehensive protocol for adrenal and thyroid health and the diagnosis and treatment of all other related conditions. For those that require more information, then the Internet, patient websites, medical websites, patient forums and libraries should be able to meet their needs, even if this requires some work.

I will now take each one of these conditions or situations in turn and discuss them very briefly.

INADEQUATE THYROID HORMONE TREATMENT DURING THE DAYTIME

Sometimes thyroid patients mistakenly believe that all they need to do to improve their cortisol levels is a properly timed and sized circadian dose of either T3 or NDT medication. The circadian dose alone may be sufficient for those patients who have partial adrenal insufficiency only, and who do not require daytime thyroid medication because their own thyroid function is adequate. However, the majority of patients using CT3M are thyroid patients and they require daytime thyroid hormone replacement. For these patients, it is important to remember that the adrenal glands need to be receiving enough thyroid hormone *over the entire day*, or CT3M will be very unlikely to work properly.

The adrenal glands appear to be quite slow to adjust to changes with respect to thyroid medication. CT3M itself can take several weeks to affect a change in cortisol and general well being. Sometimes when I am considering the adrenal glands, the image comes into my head of an ocean liner that needs constant force applied to make any noticeable change in speed or direction. If the adrenal glands do not get adequate thyroid hormones during the day, then the result is often that they cannot produce enough cortisol during the daytime - the 'ocean liner is going very slowly'. In this situation, no matter how well CT3M is applied, it is often just not sufficient to improve cortisol levels.

If cortisol levels are not improving with CT3M, then the type and dosage of thyroid hormones used during the day should be investigated. Either the dosage or the level of thyroid hormones could be too low. The type of thyroid hormones being used may not be ideal for the individual thyroid patient.

If a thyroid patient is using T4 or NDT during the daytime, then it might be worth considering the measurement of TSH, FT4, FT3 and reverse T3 levels to assess how well the T4 component is converting to T3, and whether enough of the thyroid hormones are being provided. In some cases, a proportion of the T4 component of the daytime thyroid medication might need switching to T3 to ensure that adequate levels of the biologically active T3 thyroid hormone is active within the cells. In a few cases, even apparently healthy levels of FT4 and reverse T3 levels may be a problem, and blood tests may not actually identify this. Some thyroid patients do appear to need T3 only treatment in order to feel healthier.

It is quite common to find patients who only respond to CT3M when their circadian dose is pure T3. A few may also need T3 for daytime thyroid medication. Occasionally, some thyroid patients actually do better with some T4 component in their thyroid medication in the daytime, so this may also need to be investigated if the patient is taking T3 only. There might be a need to fully investigate and do some trials with different types of thyroid medication in the daytime before making any further adjustments to the circadian dose.

It is very easy for someone to forget to put adequate focus on the daytime component of the thyroid medication. This sub-section is a reminder that for CT3M to be effective, not only does the circadian dose need to be adjusted correctly, but any daytime thyroid medication also has a role in the support of the adrenal glands (as they produce cortisol over the day, albeit at a lower level than early in the morning).

HIGHLY IRREGULAR SLEEPING / WAKING PATTERN

By *irregular sleeping / waking pattern* I mean a very broken pattern of sleep with periods of a few hours asleep followed by hours awake. Sometimes these hours are spread over twenty-four hours rather than over the eight to ten hours during which most of us attempt to sleep. This highly irregular sleep pattern may not even be the same each day. I am not discussing shift workers here, just those with very poor sleeping patterns.

Note: This is quite different to the person who goes to bed at a fixed time each night and then may have periods of time during which they are not able to sleep, or the person who may wake up during the night and not be able to sleep again.

For someone with a highly irregular sleep/wake pattern, CT3M may not be applicable because it will be impossible to determine the right time to take the circadian dose. There is a solution to this, but it can be quite difficult. The solution is to re-establish a fixed pattern of going to bed and getting up, even if periods of this time are spent awake. If this approach is taken, then CT3M could be applied and it may help. If, as a result of this, cortisol levels improve, then this should also help to re-establish a better sleep pattern, with much more restful and restorative sleep. However, for some people, re-establishing a regular pattern of going to bed and rising may be difficult to do.

LOW IRON

Iron deficiency is known to adversely affect T4 to T3 conversion, increase reverse T3 levels, and block the metabolism boosting properties of thyroid hormone. Thus, iron deficiency will result in diminished intracellular T3 levels and far less effective thyroid hormone action. Low iron was discussed in detail in Chapter 3. However, it is worth re-stating that if a thyroid patient has not done due diligence and fully checked out their iron levels (serum iron, serum ferritin, transferrin saturation %) and addressed any low levels of iron, then this can also undermine CT3M (and all thyroid hormone treatment). The full iron panel results should be obtained and checked against the levels that thyroid patient experience has found to be helpful - see Chapter 3 of this book and the *Recovering with T3* book.[RWT3 1]

METHYLATION DEFECTS

Methylation is a biochemical process or cycle that contributes to a wide range of functions in the human body:
- Detoxification.
- Immune function.
- Maintaining DNA.

- Energy production.
- Mood balancing.
- Controlling inflammation.

Through these functions, our bodies perform detoxification, rebuild damaged tissues and cope with stress of various kinds. Poor methylation function can therefore contribute to various diseases and conditions, including:

- Cardiovascular disease.
- Cancer.
- Diabetes.
- Neurological problems.
- Autism and autistic spectrum disorders (ASDs).
- Alzheimer's disease.
- Chronic fatigue syndrome.
- Fertility issues.
- Allergies.
- Gut health problems.
- Strokes.
- Depression and others chronic conditions.

Methylation is involved in almost every biochemical reaction in our body, and occurs billions of times every second in our cells. Methylation cycle issues are now starting to be recognised as important to investigate if a thyroid patient does not respond well to thyroid hormone (including CT3M).

Vitamin B6, B12, and folic acid are necessary to reduce homocysteine and keep the methylation process occurring (see sub-section on Vitamin B Complex, B12 or Folate Deficiency). When you have poor methylation your body's levels of homocysteine will elevate. Homocysteine is an amino acid that is toxic to the body. It has been seen that low levels of B vitamins can be linked to methylation issues and can raise homocysteine. By providing the right levels of B vitamins this can often decrease the homocysteine levels, and potentially reduce any conditions that are linked to the methylation issue. See also the sub-section below on Mercury / Heavy Metal Toxicity.

Genetic defects may cause this methylation process to work incorrectly. The result of this can cause what is referred to as under or over-methylation. Imbalances in the methylation process can interfere with thyroid hormone action and CT3M. This may be due to the effect on inflammation levels, the activity of the immune system or the impact on mitochondrial function that might result from a methylation problem.

Fortunately, these days there are genetic tests for methylation defects. Although the genetic defect cannot be corrected, there are diet and supplementation approaches that may be used to reverse the effects and to avoid the problems that can result. As with many of the other conditions mentioned in this chapter, it is essential to work with a competent and knowledgeable doctor to investigate possible methylation issues and then resolve them.

It is very important to investigate potential methylation issues if there has been a poor response to CT3M, as methylation issues have frequently been seen to be a source of the issues.

VITAMIN B COMPLEX, B12 OR FOLATE DEFICIENCY

These important nutrients are discussed in Chapter 3 of this book. Levels of these should be checked before starting CT3M. If they have not been evaluated however and problems persist during the application of CT3M, then they should definitely be assessed via laboratory testing. There are further tests that may be done, which are covered below.

B vitamins are known to be critical to energy production within the cells. In particular, vitamin B6, B12, B9 (folic acid, measured as *folate* in a blood test) are the rate limiting nutrients in the methylation process. If a thyroid patient does not have adequate B vitamin levels then the result can be inadequate mitochondrial function and lower cellular energy levels (ATP). This alone is enough to inhibit thyroid hormone action and CT3M.

It is common for a thyroid patient's doctor to request a B12 test. However, simply measuring B12 levels in the blood is no guarantee of adequate B12 availability and use within the cells. Often serum B12 may be high or normal when measured via a blood test. However, this can be illusory as there may not be enough vitamin B12 within our cells.

There are other ways to assess the actual availability of B12, which include laboratory testing for methylmalonic acid, M-series results via a Complete Blood Count and homocysteine.

Methylmalonic acid is the surrogate marker for B12 saturation in the cell, so this may be tested.

A complete blood count (CBC) can be helpful. In a CBC there are many useful pieces of information. Three interesting results are the MCV (mean corpuscular volume), MCH (mean corpuscular hemoglobin) and MCHC (mean corpuscular hemoglobin concentration). Collectively these are part of a CBC. They (MCV, MCH and MCHC) are called the M-series and describe the size and weight of the red blood cells.

Some doctors and naturopaths are now using slightly more helpful and practical criteria to determine if a patient has a deficiency in one or more nutrients. *Functional medicine* is one such discipline that uses tighter ranges for the results of some blood tests. Functional ranges and laboratory reference ranges are two entirely different things. A lab reference range is very broad and is obtained by pooling the results of people who may be well, but also people who may possibly be unhealthy or even ill. Functional ranges are tighter and are more useful at identifying problems. The specialty of *Functional Medicine* has established these ranges.

Functional elevations (deviations from the functional ranges) in the M-series indicate deficiencies in folic acid and B12. These functional elevations are not the same as reference ranges, and they need to be assessed and evaluated by a knowledgeable doctor or health care practitioner. However, for someone who is adequately trained, the CBC can help determine if vitamin B12 and folic acid are actually low or not, even if the blood tests of B12 and folate are normal or even high. Generally speaking, if M-series readings are near the top of the laboratory reference ranges, then this might be indicative of B12 deficiency, but seeking the help of a competent health care professional is advisable when interpreting M-series results.

There is also a relationship between the M-series and homocysteine. Homocysteine can provide some insight into B12 and folic acid levels. Sometimes the M-series can appear healthy but homocysteine may be over a certain functional level that would indicate a need for folic acid and B12. Someone trained in functional medicine can analyse the M-Series, homocysteine, vitamin B12 and folate. Simply looking at reference ranges may not be sufficient.

Evaluating the M-series, together with homocysteine and the B complex vitamin levels is a much more accurate way of evaluating B vitamin status.

The bottom line here is that the B complex vitamins, including B6, B12 and B9 (folic acid) are hugely important. They are critical to mitochondrial energy production, and therefore to thyroid hormone action and CT3M. Simplistic measurement of B12 and folate may not actually provide any real insight into the utilisation of these vitamins within our cells, and other markers need to be looked at if a true assessment of critical vitamin availability is to be performed.

The importance of these vitamins provide a rationale for supplementing B Complex and B12 at safe dosages, regardless of supposedly normal test results or situations when thorough testing is not possible.

OTHER NUTRIENT DEFICIENCIES

There are several vitamins and minerals that if low or are out of balance with other nutrients will stop thyroid hormone from being utilised inside our cells. Low magnesium, low potassium, low sodium or a potassium/sodium imbalance, low zinc or copper, or a zinc/copper imbalance, are good examples of mineral issues that may be problematic. Selenium is another nutrient that can sometimes be low and it is well-known that this can impact the conversion of T4 to T3. Vitamin D3 is also important to supplement if levels are low.[RWT3 2]

Iodine may also be valuable to assess and then supplement in some cases. Iodine is very important to the thyroid gland. It is thought that bromide and the other halides can act as toxins in the thyroid receptors and prevent them from accepting thyroid hormones. If this is the case then no amount of thyroid hormone medication will work correctly, including CT3M. There is much written on the subject of iodine and its potential role in clearing halides like bromide, fluoride and chloride that we are exposed to these days. It is beyond the scope of this book to discuss this topic in further detail. However, there are excellent books written on the subject, and there is a great deal of easily accessible information on the Internet.[3,4]

Clearly if there are digestive system issues, including a lack of gut integrity, then this can lead to malabsorption of essential vitamins and minerals. There is a sub-section later in this chapter that discusses digestive system conditions and gut integrity issues a little further.

I am no expert on vitamins and minerals, but I do believe in supplementing with a broad range of vitamins and minerals at a safe level. Thyroid patients considering investigating this area should consult their own personal physician or nutritionist for appropriate laboratory testing and guidance on a safe supplementation regime.[RWT3 2]

BLOOD SUGAR METABOLISM ISSUES

If blood sugar metabolism problems exist, then these can prevent thyroid hormones from being effective, and that of course may undermine CT3M. Chapter 7 of this book is focused on the subject of blood sugar, and *Recovering with T3* also touches on this issue.[RWT3 5]

MERCURY / HEAVY METAL TOXICITY

Mercury is a highly toxic metal that poses negative effects on human health, and in particular to the thyroid gland. Well known as a component of dental amalgam fillings, mercury contributes to thyroid disease as well as being thought to have links to low iron. Large doses of mercury are known to cause hyperthyroidism. However, lower levels of mercury in the body are thought to contribute to hypothyroidism by interfering with both the production of T4 and the conversion of T4 to the active T3. There are studies and clinical experience of some doctors indicating that mercury and toxic metal exposures appear to be a common cause of hypothyroidism.[RWT3 6]

Heavy metal toxicity (even at low levels), is thought to have an impact on the methylation system in our bodies. Disruptions to the methylation system can impact energy production and all thyroid hormone effectiveness. There have been numerous cases where thyroid patients have not responded well to thyroid hormones until they have undergone chelation of mercury or other heavy metals. It is thought that disturbances to the methylation system may be a more common issue for thyroid patients than anyone had previously considered. Methylation issues are discussed earlier in this chapter.

Thyroid patients who are continuing to experience difficulty regaining their health and who have amalgam fillings in their teeth should consider having these replaced. Amalgam filings contain mercury, and it is well known that this can have an impact on health for some people. I had my own amalgam fillings removed over 15 years ago and replaced with white, non-toxic fillings that look natural and have no heavy metal content.

There are various chelation techniques available that can assist with removing heavy metals from the body, and these can only help to promote good health.[7] Supplements such as alpha lipoic acid (mercury chelation) and DMSA (dimercaptosuccinic acid – for mercury and other heavy metals) have been used by thyroid patients with good success.

Testing for heavy metal toxicity, and any subsequent chelation to remove mercury or other heavy metals, should probably be a standard approach when thyroid hormone and CT3M do not work well. The replacement of amalgam fillings should be done before any mercury chelation is considered.

FLUORIDE TOXICITY

Even in low concentrations, fluoride is thought to impact the thyroid system in several ways by:

- Adversely affecting the manufacture of enzymes within the thyroid gland, thus slowing the production of T4 and T3 within the thyroid.
- Interacting with G proteins, and reducing the uptake of thyroid hormones into our cells.
- Reducing the pituitary gland's production of TSH.
- Affecting (as can the other halides) the thyroid receptors in the cell nuclei and mitochondria, thus reducing the binding of thyroid hormones within our cells.

Many health professionals are concerned about the addition of fluoride to our water supplies, and the many other sources of fluoride and halides in our environment. It is well known that the incidence of hypothyroidism is increasing. The use of fluoride in our water and other products is something we should all be concerned about.

Fluoride is also known to displace iodine in our body. It was recently pointed out that iodine deficiency is growing worldwide. In the UK, there are areas that are now iodine deficient. In a recent study, it was shown that 40% of pregnant women in the Tayside region of Scotland were deficient by at least half of the iodine required for a normal pregnancy. A relatively high level of missing, decayed or filled teeth was observed in this non-fluoridated area. It has been suggested that the iodine deficiency in this area was causing early hypothyroidism, which interferes with the health of teeth. In areas that are fluoridated, any existing iodine deficiency would potentially be made significantly worse.

Some thyroid patients have had success with iodine therapy. As mentioned within the Other Nutrient Deficiencies sub-section, one of the potential benefits ascribed to the use of iodine is that it may help to detoxify the thyroid hormone receptors of halides such as bromide and fluoride.

SEX HORMONE IMBALANCES

Sex hormone imbalances can occur in both men and women.[RWT3 8] However, it is quite common for women to have an imbalance in oestrogen and progesterone, frequently with progesterone being too low. This *oestrogen dominance* may lower the production and action of thyroid hormones. This may be one reason why it is so common for hypothyroidism to make its first appearance when a woman begins to approach the menopause.

It is important for women to have at least progesterone and estradiol tested (via a blood test) between days 19 and 23 of their cycle if they still have a menstrual cycle (any day of the month if they do not). Ideally, DHEAS, testosterone and sex hormone binding globulin (SHBG) will also be tested. For men, the most important sex hormone tests are total testosterone and SHBG, but free testosterone and estradiol may also provide additional information.

For women, progesterone should ideally be in a 300:1 ratio to estradiol once these two have been converted into the same units (they are often presented in different units of measurement). Deficiency in progesterone often needs to be dealt with, as this will correct oestrogen dominance, improve many menopausal symptoms like sweats and mood swings, and help to reverse or manage osteoporosis.

Correcting oestrogen dominance can also be a critical part of making thyroid hormones work more effectively, and this of course extends to the effectiveness of CT3M if it is being used. These days, natural bio-identical progesterone cream is easily obtained, and it may also have the potential to help stabilise adrenal function.

Sex hormones should certainly be investigated if thyroid hormone and CT3M are not working as expected. It is important to work with a knowledgeable doctor to ensure that sex hormones are only replaced if needed.

UNDIAGNOSED HYPOPITUITARISM OR HPA AXIS PROBLEMS

The hypothalamic-pituitary-adrenal axis (HPA or HTPA axis) is a complex set of direct influences and feedback interactions among the hypothalamus, the pituitary, and the adrenal glands. The interactions among these organs constitute the HPA axis, which is a major part of the neuroendocrine system. The HPA axis controls reactions to stress and regulates many body processes: including digestion, the immune system, mood and emotions, sexuality and energy storage and expenditure.

Via the HPA axis, ACTH is produced by the pituitary gland. ACTH is transported in the blood to the adrenal cortex of the adrenal gland, where it rapidly stimulates biosynthesis of corticosteroids such as cortisol from cholesterol. Cortisol is a major stress hormone and has effects on many tissues in the body, including the brain. Cortisol and other glucocorticoids in turn act back on the hypothalamus and pituitary (to suppress ACTH production) in a negative feedback cycle. This is why taking any form of steroids often results in suppressing the stimulation from the pituitary, making the adrenal cortex more sluggish than it was to begin with.

Issues with the HPA axis can also result in low growth hormone level, which can produce problems for the thyroid patient. It is beyond the scope of *The CT3M Handbook* to explore this area, but I do know of one or two thyroid patients who have eventually gone on to have growth hormone tested, found it was low and then gained improvements in their health after beginning regular injections with growth hormone. Clearly, a very experienced and knowledgeable doctor would need to be found to work with during the diagnostic and treatment process. Note: growth hormone usage can actually increase cortisol needs in some people.

If the pituitary gland is not producing enough ACTH (or one or more other of its stimulatory hormones) then this is referred to as hypopituitarism. In this chapter, our concern is primarily with the production of ACTH, because if ACTH is not being produced (as often or at the level it is required), then cortisol levels will be too low.

If there is any suspicion that the HPA axis might be a factor in continuing partial adrenal insufficiency, and CT3M does not appear to be helping, then further laboratory testing might be advisable. The patient should consult their doctor or endocrinologist and discuss this fully. In some cases the level of ACTH might be measured. This may often be inconclusive as ACTH is pulsatile in nature and fluctuates significantly during the day. A more conclusive test for hypopituitarism, or a HPA axis problem that has pituitary gland involvement, is the *Insulin Tolerance Test* (ITT) that is described in Chapter 7 of this book. The ITT is considered by many to be the gold standard test for hypopituitarism, as it creates the specific condition of low blood sugar, which the pituitary gland should respond to by producing ACTH in order to raise blood cortisol, and thus raise blood sugar once again. In addition to these laboratory tests, the patient's doctor may also wish to rule out any physical problems by performing an MRI of the thyroid patient's pituitary gland and hypothalamus.

If the HPA axis is considered to be a potential issue, and the thyroid patient's doctor wishes to avoid prescribing steroids, then there are other approaches that might still offer some help.

There are glandular products that have had their actual pituitary and hypothalamic hormone content (like ACTH) removed, and these may be of benefit. This leaves the other nutrients and co-factors that may enable the thyroid patient's pituitary and hypothalamus to function better. The idea behind products like these is to support the proper function of the HPA axis and then, after a period of time, to wean the glandulars. This is not the same as providing the actual pituitary or hypothalamus hormones. Some doctors in the USA have found value in the use of products like this.

I am aware that a few doctors in the USA are working on methods designed to support improved neurotransmitter function, as this can have a bearing on the HPA axis. I know very little about this at the present time, and it is not an approach that is being widely used. However, it is very intriguing and may offer a breakthrough for those few thyroid patients with issues in the HPA axis area.

In Chapters 25 and 29 of *Recovering with T3*, I briefly mention a drug called low dose naltrexone (LDN). Naltrexone is an opioid antagonist that has been used and approved to treat opioid addiction and alcohol addiction - at high doses. When naltrexone is taken in low doses, it is known as low dose naltrexone or LDN. LDN has been shown by researchers to work in a different way to naltrexone. LDN is believed to stimulate the production of more endorphins, which modulates the immune system and re-balances any excessive immune system responses through its effect on opioid receptors. Low dose naltrexone (LDN) is currently being used to treat some autoimmune diseases.

LDN is also thought to reduce the production of pro-inflammatory cytokines, which in turn may help thyroid hormone action. There is also some evidence that LDN appears to help improve cortisol levels in some patients. The belief is that this may be via some interaction in the HPA axis, but it might also be due to its effect in lowering some cytokines. More research is needed in this area, but certainly LDN is an option that ought to be considered by the patient's doctor if HPA axis issues or partial adrenal insufficiency continue to provide cause for concern.

I have talked to thyroid patients who have had to lower their T3 or NDT medication after starting to use LDN. I suspect this may be due to improved cortisol due to the action of LDN. This is one reason why I think LDN is a viable option to consider if CT3M has not been sufficient to correct a thyroid patient's adrenal issues. See Chapter 20 for more on LDN.

CT3M will not work for everyone of course. In the case where there appears to be a HPA axis issue that does not respond to any corrective approach attempted, then a patient's doctor may have no other solution than the use of adrenal steroids or adrenal glandulars to replace the missing adrenal hormones.

UNDIAGNOSED ADDISON'S DISEASE

This sub-section is here for completeness only, as Addison's disease has already been discussed in Chapter 3 of this book. Clearly, if Addison's disease is something that the patient and their doctor are concerned could be a possibility, then a Synacthen test (ACTH stimulation test) should be arranged if one has not already been done. In addition, the main adrenal autoantibodies could also be tested, as it is frequently an autoimmune attack that causes Addison's disease. The main adrenal autoantibodies are listed in Chapter 3 of this book.

USE OF ANTI-DEPRESSANTS

It is well known that anti-depressants may have a deleterious effect on cortisol and on FT4 to FT3 conversion. Long-term anti-depressant use is something to be avoided if possible. **However, any changes to anti-depressant medication should be discussed with a patient's own family doctor. Depression is very serious, and its effects can be devastating. Consequently, great care must be taken with any changes to anti-depressant medication.**

The use of anti-depressants is known to interfere with the hypothalamic pituitary adrenal axis (HPA axis). Some anti-depressants have a profound effect on the HPA axis. It can also take a long time to wean some anti-depressants, and the impact on the HPA axis sometimes continues for months (or even years) after the weaning has been completed, as the withdrawal effects can be significant.

Consequently, in the case of a thyroid patient who is taking or has recently taken anti-depressants, great patience may be required. From the experience of patients who have been through this process of weaning and withdrawal from antidepressants, the types of problems that are typically seen are:

- High sensitivity to thyroid hormone (often with rapid heart rate, even with very small doses of thyroid hormone).
- Difficulty in raising FT3 levels on NDT.
- Difficulty in tolerating NDT or T3 medication.
- Low cortisol levels and symptoms of partial adrenal insufficiency.

This is a really hard class of problem to solve, and it requires a great deal of patience on the part of both patient and doctor as the withdrawal process continues.

In one piece of research, it was pointed out that anti-depressants often raise the level of the neurotransmitter serotonin.[9] The body attempts to combat the elevated serotonin by raising cortisol and adrenaline. However, any short-term benefit that this effect may have may be followed in time by adrenal exhaustion. Over time, as partial adrenal insufficiency begins to take place and cortisol levels fall, the patient may experience fatigue. It is reported that many SSRI users have fatigue symptoms and it may take a long time for this to correct after the anti-depressants are no longer being used.

In another recent research study, it was shown that patients using tricyclic anti-depressants had alterations in the HPA axis. Furthermore, the study showed that those that had a lower rise in cortisol when they woke up had the strongest reductions in salivary cortisol.[10]

I have heard reports from a large number of thyroid patients over the past year whose partial adrenal insufficiency appears to have developed after the use of anti-depressants. Many of these have reported such high sensitivity to all types of thyroid medication that they were not able to tolerate enough thyroid medication to resolve their hypothyroidism. This has made it difficult for them and their medical practitioners to implement CT3M. In some cases CT3M has not worked at all for some thyroid patients who have used anti-depressants for many years.

It appears to be clear that the use of antidepressants can affect the HPA axis. It may take considerable time after the weaning of these medications for the HPA axis, and ultimately the adrenals, to have a chance of responding as they are supposed to do.

However, some patients do need to use anti-depressants. Any weaning of them

should be done with the full involvement of the patient's own doctor, and after the thyroid patient has carried out their own research on the particular anti-depressant that they are using.

LOWERED CORTISOL DUE TO THE UNHELPFUL SIDE EFFECT OF SOME NUTRIENTS

Over the past year, many people have contacted me and informed me that some minerals, herbs and other medications or products that thyroid patients use may actually have the side effect of lowering cortisol. I don't know the mechanism involved in most of these cases, but it is useful to be aware that some minerals, herbs and drugs can have this effect on cortisol. Some even depress cortisol levels the day after taking them, and should be avoided for those with low morning cortisol.

A few of the main products that thyroid patients have told me about are:

- Zinc.
- Phosphatidyl serine.
- Seriphos.
- Holy basil.
- Valerian.
- Melatonin.
- Tryptophan.
- Antidepressants (see previous sub-section).

The above are just the most well-known products that are known to have a depressive effect on cortisol levels. There may be other herbs, medications or nutrients that also do this. It is advisable for thyroid patients to do their own research on products they are using if they already have partial adrenal insufficiency.

DIGESTIVE SYSTEM CONDITIONS OR GUT INTEGRITY ISSUES

Poor gut health can impact thyroid function. Gut health is now known to be a factor in the start of Hashimoto's thyroiditis. Conversely, it is also well known that poor thyroid hormone levels can lead to gut problems like bloating, inflammation and leaky gut.

Focusing on gut health will be a major benefit to any thyroid patient and may well be the key to calming down their immune system.

Hippocrates said, "All disease begins in the gut". It appears he may have been on to something.

The gut has multiple functions:

1. It is where our food is digested, nutrients are absorbed and indigestible waste is removed from our body.

2. It is designed to prevent substances that we are not meant to digest from getting inside our bloodstream and to the rest of the body.

3. It plays host to 70% of our immune system tissue. This part of our immune system is called GALT (gut-associated lymphoid tissue). The GALT is made up from several types of lymphoid tissues that store immune cells, such as T & B lymphocytes. These carry out attacks and produce antibodies against antigens, which are molecules recognized by the immune system as dangerous.

4. It also performs a critical role in the conversion of FT4 to FT3.

The health of the gut may be viewed as linked to the health of the gut flora and the gut wall/gut barrier. The gut flora is integral to the health of the gut itself. The gut contains over ten times the number of bacteria than the number of human cells in the body! This is estimated to be over 100 trillion microorganisms! In a way we are made from more non-human microorganisms than human tissue! The gut flora promote healthy function in the gut, form a key part of our immune system and protect us from infection and hostile attack from non-friendly microorganisms. An imbalance in the gut flora has been linked to diseases like autism, depression, autoimmune conditions, diabetes and inflammatory conditions of the bowel. An imbalance of the gut flora is sometimes referred to as *intestinal dysbiosis*.

The balance of the gut flora can be damaged by various things, such as antibiotic use, diets that are high in carbohydrates and sugar, diets high in wheat and industrial seed oil, birth control pills, stress or NSAID use.

The gut wall or gut barrier provides a tube through which undigested food may pass while it is being digested. It provides the home for the gut flora, and whilst it remains healthy it prevents large protein molecules from passing out of the gut and into the bloodstream. If the gut barrier becomes permeable, it is known as *leaky gut syndrome*. If the health of the gut flora is maintained, then leaky gut syndrome should never occur. However, if the balance of the gut flora is compromised and leaky gut syndrome does develop, then many things can go wrong.

When the gut becomes permeable, as in *leaky gut syndrome*, proteins that are not broken down sufficiently, or ones that should not be absorbed at all, may leak through the gut lining and into the bloodstream. When this happens the immune system senses these substances that should not be there and attempts to attack them. Research has shown that this is a likely mechanism in the development of autoimmune diseases like Hashimoto's thyroiditis.

It is also worth noting that someone could have leaky gut syndrome without any symptoms that they can detect within their own gut. Leaky gut can cause problems with skin conditions, depression, autoimmune conditions, type 1 diabetes and several other conditions. Wheat and other grains that contain gluten are thought to be a major factor in the development of leaky gut syndrome.

If someone develops leaky gut syndrome, then the inflammation and excess immune system activity that results may leave the patient with one or more of the following:

- Fatigue.
- Brain fog.
- Depression.
- Skin irritations/conditions.
- Metabolic issues perhaps leading to obesity.
- Asthma.
- Allergies.
- Autoimmune diseases.

These can be indistinguishable from some symptoms that patients with thyroid disease often have. For this reason, a thyroid patient may go for a considerable time before they discover that they have a serious issue with the health of their gut. Some people may never realise that this is one major source of their health problems.

Let me now discuss some of the relationships between the health of the gut and thyroid hormone action, as it is these that caused me to add gut integrity problems to the list of conditions that might disrupt CT3M and thyroid hormone action.

Good thyroid hormone levels have been shown to protect the gut lining. In studies of gastric ulcers, low T3 and T4 levels have been found, and high levels of rT3 have been detected.

The mechanism of conversion of T4 to T3 is greatly dependant on liver and gut health. Much of this conversion takes place within the liver, but it may be surprising to learn that around 20% of the T4 converted to T3 takes place in the gut. It is very important to appreciate how critical it is to have healthy gut and liver function.

In a thyroid patient with an immune system that is overactive due to autoimmunity, the raised levels of cytokines (immune system modulators) can provoke a rise in the cytokine IL17, which is known to damage the gut lining. Cytokines may also be raised due to gluten and other food sensitivities, and these cytokines can also cause a rise in IL17. Elevated cortisol from stress responses may also compromise the intestinal lining integrity, as can the use of adrenal steroids and adrenal glandulars. This further illustrates the importance of focusing on maintaining optimal gut and liver function.

An imbalance in the gut flora (intestinal dysbiosis) reduces the conversion of T4 thyroid hormone into the biologically active T3. In addition to this, inflammation that arises out of dysbiosis creates more demand for cortisol, which is needed to dampen down the inflammation. Increased cortisol may impact thyroid hormone action if it rises beyond the normal level for the individual, and this in turn can raise rT3 levels and decrease T3 levels.

There are also studies that show that the cell walls of some pathogenic bacteria can affect thyroid hormones by reducing active levels of T3, blocking thyroid receptors, increasing rT3, decreasing TSH and helping to create the conditions for Hashimoto's thyroiditis.

Low thyroid hormone is also known to reduce stomach acid levels. Low stomach acid (hypochlorhydria) in turn allows more bad bacteria to flourish, increases gut permeability and inflammation. There are connections between gastritis and autoimmune conditions. Low thyroid hormone often causes the gut to slow down, and this can impair the clearance of hormones like oestrogen, which can also impact thyroid hormone action further. Constipation will also increase inflammation and the risk of further bacteria imbalance and poor absorption of nutrients.

A compromised gut or low stomach acid may also result in low blood sugar, and it may well restrict the availability of important nutrients like iron, B12, magnesium, B vitamins etc. that in turn can affect CT3M and thyroid hormone action.

A heightened immune system response to pathogens and large protein molecules that may cross into the blood due to leaky gut is linked to autoimmune thyroid disease. It is known that some immune system chemicals called cytokines can impact the action of thyroid hormone within the cells. This can require more thyroid hormone to be present in the cells in order to maintain adequate thyroid hormone action. In some cases, the presence of high levels of cytokines may require thyroid hormone treatments like NDT or T3, in order to overcome the effects of the cytokines. Action should also be taken to calm down the immune system. The removal of grains that contain gluten from the diet (like wheat) can often be extremely helpful. The removal of dairy and soy products may also benefit some people.

Based on all the above, it should be clear that repairing a leaky gut may be an essential step in the recovery from thyroid and adrenal issues for many thyroid patients. I cannot stress this last point enough - it is crucial.

Even though the immune system attacks the thyroid gland, Hashimoto's thyroiditis is a disease of the immune system, not the thyroid gland. If the immune dysfunction is not corrected, then thyroid medications and CT3M will not work well. Healing the gut is often a critical part in dealing with the immune system dysfunction - even if the thyroid patient is not aware of any obvious digestive system symptoms!

There are helpful approaches to <u>heal the gut</u>. To have a healthy gut, you need good levels of thyroid hormones and especially the biologically active thyroid hormone T3. You also won't get thyroid hormone action to be effective without a healthy gut, so simply taking the right thyroid hormones, at the right dosage, may not be sufficient.

To begin the journey to heal the gut, the sources of imbalances to the gut flora and damage to the intestinal barrier must be removed. Then healthy gut flora must be restored. Typical steps necessary to restore gut health include:

- Removal of all food toxins from the diet - especially gluten containing grains like wheat, or any other food types that are clearly causing sensitivities. Dairy and soy products often have to be removed from the diet too.

- Address any low stomach acid issue if it is present by using an appropriate nutritional supplement (low thyroid hormone levels or low cortisol can also cause low stomach acid).

- Take a high-quality, multi-species probiotic to replace the friendly bacteria.

- Treat any intestinal pathogens (such as parasites) that may be present.

- Use a diet that is designed to improve gut health, e.g. GAPS or Paleo, or the exclusion of the irritating food types (as already discussed).

- Use supplements that are known to aid gut healing. A competent naturopath or doctor used to working in this area should be able to advise on a suitable product(s) or supplements.

- The use of immune system modulating supplements can also help. Some which have been found to be effective are: fish oil, vitamin D3 and glutathione.

- The immune system produces various types of cytokines as part of the immune system response. Two groups of cytokines are known as TH1 and TH2. If one or both of these groups are out of balance, then they may be corrected using dietary changes and supplementation. Datis Kharrazian has written an excellent book on this topic[11]. It is possible to have tests to determine whether a thyroid patient has raised TH1 or TH2 cytokines. There are products that will push the TH1 TH2 pathways in either direction, thus managing the immune system.

- Implement changes to lower stress.

- Read further on the subject of gut health and dietary changes[12, 13, 14, 15,16]

A thyroid patient may have some or no obvious gut symptoms, but the health of their gut barrier and their gut flora may be a huge contributory factor in whether they are successfully responding to thyroid hormones and CT3M.

CHRONIC INFLAMMATION ISSUES

Inflammation is a normal physiological response of the human body. It is designed to protect us and remove harmful stimuli, which might include irritants, damaged cells or pathogens. Inflammation also begins the process of healing.

When a harmful stimulus affects the human body there is an inflammatory response. If the harmful stimulus is serious enough, the inflammatory response will be noticeable. This is called *acute inflammation*. The acute inflammation response indicates that the body is trying to heal itself, and this is a fundamental part of our immune system. The common features of acute inflammation are:

- Pain in the inflamed area. This is often caused by the release of chemicals to that area. These chemicals stimulate nerve endings and make the area painful.
- Redness. Due to more blood being present in capillaries in the region.
- Immobility. The muscle or joint may lose some movement or function.
- Swelling. This is caused by fluid build up.
- Heat. This is for the same reason as the redness in the area.

Acute inflammation starts rapidly and quickly becomes severe. Signs and symptoms are only present for a few days, but in some cases they may persist for a few weeks.

This inflammatory response to injury, or attack by bacteria or other pathogens, is necessary and helpful. However, sometimes inflammation can cause further inflammation; it can become a vicious circle in which more inflammation is created in response to the existing inflammation. When this vicious circle is entered and the inflammation becomes long term then it is referred to as *chronic inflammation*, which can last for several months and even years.

Chronic inflammation can result from several factors. It may be that the body has failed to remove the cause of the original acute inflammation. Autoimmunity may have developed in response to a self-antigen, which results in the immune system constantly attacking healthy cells. Some chronic irritant may continue to exist in the body. There are many diseases that include the presence of chronic inflammation. Some examples are: chronic peptic ulcers, asthma, rheumatoid arthritis and inflammatory bowel diseases.

Our wounds and infections would not heal without inflammation. However, chronic inflammation can eventually cause several diseases and conditions. **We also know that the presence of chronic inflammation appears to interfere with thyroid hormone action, and in some cases it may cause CT3M to be far less effective than it should be.** The exact mechanism of this interference to thyroid hormone is not fully understood. However, we already know that some immune system chemicals can block the action of thyroid hormones within the cells, e.g. some cytokines are known to do this. So, it is entirely plausible that chronic inflammation would make CT3M less effective than it should be.

In thyroid patients with Hashimoto's thyroiditis we already know that there is an active autoimmune response in progress. Consequently, it is important to do whatever can be done to lower the level of this response.[RWT3 17]

If chronic inflammation is suspected, then there are various laboratory tests that may help to confirm this. These include:

- C- reactive protein test (CRP).
- Erythrocyte sedimentation rate test (ESR).
- White cell blood count.
- Serum ferritin (ferritin is often high in the presence of chronic inflammation).

If chronic inflammation is present, and the cause of this inflammation is still present, then it should be treated. In many thyroid patients the source of the inflammation may be the gluten-containing foods still in the diet, and potentially some other food sensitivity (dairy products or soy for instance).

After prolonged hypothyroidism, some thyroid patients may have developed an imbalance in the microorganisms in the gut, which can lead to inflammation. Focusing on the health of the gut may be one of the single most effective strategies a thyroid patient can adopt to resolve inflammation and other issues.

There are various supplements that thyroid patients have found to be of help in reducing inflammation. These include:

- Krill oil.
- Colostrum.
- Omega 3 (fish oil).
- Herbs such as turmeric/ginger.
- Astaxanthin.

The use of low dose naltrexone (LDN) has in some cases been seen to be helpful because LDN can modulate the immune system and, in doing so, reduce inflammation.

The use of supplements or medications (like LDN) should be discussed with the patient's own medical practitioner. See Chapter 20 for more about LDN.

LOW LEVELS OF RELATED ADRENAL HORMONES

In some cases, thyroid patients have found that their issues have been due to low levels of one or more other hormones. Hormones like pregnenolone, DHEA or progesterone may need to be supplemented before CT3M will work successfully. However, it is important to work closely with a knowledgeable doctor, using laboratory testing to reach this type of conclusion and then to deal with any deficiency correctly.

Pregnenolone is called the mother of all steroid hormones. It is the precursor of female hormones such as oestrogen and progesterone; mineral corticoids such as aldosterone; glucocorticoids such as cortisol; and androgens such as testosterone. Pregnenolone is therefore known as a pro-hormone. During periods of stress, the output of adrenal steroids such as cortisol will increase, which will put a great demand on pregnenolone production. This may lead to pregnenolone deficiency, which in turn may lead to a reduction of both cortisol and aldosterone. This deficiency is sometimes referred to as *pregnenolone steal*.

Taking pregnenolone for partial adrenal insufficiency may not be straightforward, as some patients experience a benefit from it and others feel worse when pregnenolone is supplemented. Pregnenolone is converted in the body to progesterone. Pregnenolone is also converted into DHEA, which may convert into androstendione, testosterone and oestrogens. Consequently, it is very important to work with a doctor who understands and has experience with the use of pregnenolone. Pregnenolone use is sometimes advised against for those with a history of seizures.

If DHEA is found to be low, then it may also need to be supplemented. Progesterone may also be an issue and ought to be tested and supplemented if low. Please refer to the discussion on sex hormones earlier in the chapter for more information.

MITOCHONDRIAL DISEASE OR ISSUES

If mitochondrial issues exist, then CT3M could easily be prevented from working. The mitochondria are the entities within our cells that make ATP. This topic is covered in Chapter 7.

The mitochondria use various co-factors in the production of ATP. These include: L-carnitine, coenzyme Q-10, NADH, B complex vitamins, lipoic acid, magnesium and various other nutrients.

Coenzyme Q10 is incorporated into the mitochondria of our cells where it facilitates the transformation of fats and sugars into energy. There is scientific evidence that shows Co-Q10's ability to restore mitochondrial function, which in turn has a positive effect on the health of the patient.

There are two forms of Co-Q10: Ubiquinol and Ubiquinone. Ubiquinol is the biologically superior form of Co-Q10. Some doctors are beginning to routinely use 200 mg of Co-Q10 per day with thyroid patients, as this is thought to strengthen the mitochondria. There are many scientific papers that can easily be found on the Internet that point to the links between Co-Q10 and mitochondrial health.

Whilst congenital mitochondrial lesions are rare, acquired mitochondrial dysfunction is common. Dr. Sarah Myhill often runs a Mitochondrial Function Test with ME patients. She has told me that mitochondrial dysfunction is seen frequently in these patients. I personally suspect that mitochondrial issues are more common than many people and doctors suspect. For those thyroid patients who still struggle with achieving good health after all else has been tried, and other issues (like low cortisol, low iron, blood sugar issues etc) have been resolved, then using Co-Q10 and other mitochondrial co-factors may be an approach that offers some value. As ever, working with a knowledgeable and competent medical physician is important.

There are medical tests that can be carried out by a few specialist centres to assess the performance of the mitochondria. The test results can be used to determine which of a possible set of supplements might be most beneficial. However, if all else has failed, low ATP production may be investigated as a possible cause of poor response to thyroid hormone or CT3M.

IMMUNE SYSTEM HYPER-ACTIVITY

This small sub-section overlaps with previous sub-sections including: *Other Nutrient Deficiencies*; *Digestive System Conditions or Gut Integrity Issues*; and *Chronic Inflammation Issues*.

If the thyroid patient's immune system is overactive, then the effect of this can be to block the effectiveness of thyroid hormone, which may include the action of CT3M. The important thing in the first instance is to remove any remaining causes of immune system activity. For Hashimoto's thyroiditis patients, this frequently necessitates the exclusion of gluten from the diet, and may also require the exclusion of dairy and soy. For patients with an overactive immune system, it may mean the treatment of a specific medical condition or disease that has immune system involvement. For instance, the removal of any other foods that cause issues to the individual, a gut repair programme, or a better approach to dealing with stress. I also discuss supplements that can help to down-regulate the immune system in the sub-section above on gut integrity issues.

In addition to the basic approaches just mentioned, there are other techniques that may be worthwhile investigating.

Some thyroid patients have achieved success with Iodine Therapy. One of the potential benefits that is ascribed to the use of iodine is that it may help to detoxify the thyroid hormone receptors of halides like bromide and fluoride.

Low dose naltexone (LDN) has been found to be useful by some thyroid patients. Apart from calming the immune system, LDN is thought by some to help to rebalance the HPA axis, and I know of some patients who have had improved twenty-four hour adrenal saliva tests as a result of LDN use. This is definitely an approach that should be considered by the thyroid patient and their doctor after the more standard approaches have been attempted.

Supplementation with vitamin D3 has been seen to be helpful for thyroid patients, especially those with low vitamin D and autoimmune thyroiditis.[RWT3 2]

The supplement Berberine has become of interest also, and appears to be of help to some people. Berberine is an alkaloid that is present in a number of plants. It is thought to be of benefit through lowering the level of pro-inflammatory cytokines in the body.

SOME BACTERIAL OR VIRAL INFECTIONS

The presence of other diseases may undermine CT3M. These diseases may be known about by the patient and their doctor, or may be as yet undiagnosed. This list may not be complete, but the diseases that are known to undermine thyroid hormone action and CT3M (that have not been mentioned elsewhere in the chapter) are:

- Lyme disease.
- Re-activated EBV (Epstein Barr Virus), which can be common for hypothyroid patients under stress.
- Other bacterial, viral or fungal infections that are causing the patient's immune system to be very active.

... I expect more will be added to this list over time.

Some infections are hard to diagnose and each infection needs the appropriate treatment. Working with a knowledgeable doctor for diagnosis and treatment of infections like these is essential.

FINAL THOUGHTS

I wrote this chapter because for some patients, CT3M does not work as well as it should. In a few cases, CT3M does not work at all. Many of the causes of CT3M failure are actually resolvable if the specific problem can be identified. Some causes may not be resolvable, and in some cases (even after much investigation) then no answers may be found and CT3M may be abandoned.

For those thyroid patients who do have problems getting a good response to CT3M, this chapter provides the starting list of ideas that may be discussed between the patient and their own doctor.

CT3M works well for many. However, for those that it does not help, this chapter should provide a good starting point for further investigation.

Much credit should go to the T3CM Forum administrators, and Dawn Vo in particular, for investigating the links between methylation defects/heavy metal toxicity and the poor response to CT3M in some patients. I expect more will be learned about these and other issues in time.

Chapter 9

When to Begin CT3M

There is no right answer to this, as it depends on the thyroid patient's problems and how their doctor wants to proceed.

The thyroid patient may have recently been diagnosed with hypothyroidism and partial adrenal insufficiency. More likely, they have been on thyroid medication for some time and they or their doctor have realised that there is a problem with low cortisol.

The thyroid patient may be using T4 (levothyroxine), or NDT or T3, or some combination of these. Some thyroid patients are already on a full replacement dose of T3 or NDT when they discover or suspect that they have a low cortisol problem.

They may have known about the partial adrenal insufficiency for some time, and their doctor may even have been trying to alleviate the symptoms through the use of adrenal glandulars or steroids like hydrocortisone. Some thyroid patients may have been in this latter category for some years and have only recently heard about the existence of CT3M.

In the case of someone who is still very under-medicated on NDT, T3, or even T4 medication, then it may be desirable to attempt to raise the thyroid medication in order to see if the partial adrenal insufficiency simply corrects once a more appropriate level of thyroid medication is in place. For a thyroid patient using T4 medication only, a more successful treatment may require the change of thyroid medication from T4 to something more effective like NDT or T3 over the day. These options should be discussed between the patient and their own doctor. If the adrenal issues are minor, then the use of CT3M may be delayed until there has been an attempt to optimise the daytime thyroid medication.

Some thyroid patients have extremely poor adrenal function. If there is no hypopituitarism, Addison's disease, serious blood sugar or iron issues present, then starting CT3M alongside the start of using any thyroid hormone may be the best approach. Some individuals have done this with good success. In fact, some thyroid patients have such adrenal weakness that only the use of CT3M allows them to build up tolerance for thyroid hormone.

With very low cortisol, the attempt to optimise thyroid medication can cause various problems. The problems may range from a virtually negligible response to any thyroid hormone increases, to the very rapid heart rate brought on by adrenaline release (this latter response is common, and is described by some thyroid patients as a *sensitivity to thyroid medications,* but it is really just adrenaline and not genuine sensitivity). In these situations, it is common to make the circadian dose the largest dose of T3 or NDT because of the lack of tolerance to anything other than tiny daytime doses of thyroid medication until cortisol levels are improved.

For thyroid patients with clearly diagnosed partial adrenal insufficiency, then the immediate use of CT3M is often the best approach, even when someone has recently been prescribed NDT or T3 medication.

To summarise, CT3M can be applied at any time in the dosage management process depending on the needs of the thyroid patient. There is no fixed stage or optimal time to begin CT3M. However, as mentioned earlier in Chapter 3, it is important to be sure CT3M is relevant.

Chapter 10

The Use of Adrenal Adaptogens

An adaptogen is a plant or herbal extract, which may be used to lower or raise our adrenal response. They are naturally occurring substances, taken by thyroid patients with the objective of evening out adrenal response and helping patients to rebalance adrenal steroids like cortisol.

Adrenal adaptogens include:

- Ashwagandha (often used to modulate cortisol, by raising it a little when it is needed over the day and lowering it a little when required).
- Eleuthero (this can help thyroid patients cope with stress and boost the immune system).
- Ginseng (used to stimulate the adrenals to produce more cortisol, but not in the evening as it can prevent sleep).
- Holy Basil (often used to lower cortisol when it is too high).
- Rhodiola Rosea (helps to recover from stress and can raise cortisol levels).
- Phosphatidyl serine (sometimes referred to as PS. This is often used to help the thyroid patient reduce high evening / night cortisol and aid sleep. This adaptogen may be found in products that combine herbs like Adrenal Calm. PS is sometimes combined with zinc in the evening to lower evening / night cortisol).

.... There are many more adrenal adaptogens.

A twenty-four hour adrenal saliva test provides the most useful insight into the level of free cortisol (bio-available cortisol) over the day. Four results of free cortisol measured in saliva show free cortisol soon after getting up in the morning, late morning, late afternoon and evening. This profile of free cortisol is only currently available from an adrenal saliva test, as blood testing of cortisol does not measure free or biologically active cortisol levels. If the profile of free cortisol does not follow the expected healthy pattern, then adrenal adaptogens may help.

If there is only very mild low cortisol at some points, then adrenal adaptogens alone may be sufficient to correct this and help the thyroid patient recover from stress, i.e. CT3M may not be needed at all.

Where the profile of cortisol over the day shows low cortisol at some points, then an appropriately selected adrenal adaptogen(s) taken at the right time may help the adrenal glands to recover when combined with CT3M use.

Alternatively, if the profile of cortisol shows cortisol that is higher than the healthy level at some points, then the correctly chosen adrenal adaptogen(s) can be of great help in lowering the cortisol level. However, it should be taken at the right time in relation to this raised cortisol.

The specific use of each adrenal adaptogen is beyond the scope of this book. However, it is important to introduce them here as they are frequently extremely helpful when combined with good nutrition and stress management techniques. There is a wealth of information on the Internet regarding adrenal adaptogens, and increasingly doctors and naturopaths recommend their use (perhaps more so in the USA than in other countries, but this may slowly be changing).

SECTION 2

THE CIRCADIAN T3 METHOD

Chapter 11

The Circadian T3 Method (CT3M)

This chapter describes the basic process of applying the Circadian T3 Method (CT3M). Subsequent chapters within this section discuss aspects of CT3M that thyroid patients and their doctors sometimes need detailed information about. Consequently, it will be necessary to read all the chapters in this section to gain a comprehensive and deep knowledge of CT3M.

WHAT IF ADRENAL GLANDULARS OR STEROIDS ARE BEING USED

If a thyroid patient is already using adrenal glandulars or adrenal steroids before starting CT3M, then a decision needs to be made to either leave these in place and wean them during CT3M (the typical approach), or to wean them before commencing CT3M. The thyroid patient and their doctor will need to discuss which option to use. I have mentioned several times that some patients will need to take adrenal steroids due to diagnosed medical conditions like Addison's disease, hypopituitarism or inflammatory conditions. I won't expand on that here as it is covered in other chapters e.g. Chapter 3.

PRACTICALITIES OF THE CIRCADIAN DOSE - MEDICATION, ALARMS, WATER ETC

In CT3M, I have termed the early morning dose of thyroid medication the *circadian dose*. The circadian dose of T3 or NDT should be prepared beforehand (for instance, just before going to bed), and put in some kind of small container that makes it very easy to find in the dark. I personally use one of those tiny milk cartons that you get in cafes, which are used to put small measure of milk into coffee or tea. Other patients use eggcups, or other small household containers.

Some water in a glass within hand reach is also a good idea. Washing the circadian dose down with a mouthful of water ensures that it all reaches the stomach in one go - which is the best way to achieve swift absorption of the circadian dose.

An alarm clock, watch alarm or mobile phone alarm should be set to the time of the circadian dose and placed next to the bed. For those that need to make very little noise in order to not wake others, then there are various options. A vibration alarm could be used and placed under the pillow. Alternatively, two alarms could be used with the first being a quiet one and the second one being a louder alarm set 10 minutes later. I have always used the two-alarm approach, and I just turn the louder one off once I hear the watch alarm.

It is not a good idea to sit up and put a light on as this can cause the individual to wake up properly and not be able to sleep again.

So, with all of this next to the bed, the thyroid patient should be able to hear the alarm, turn it off and take the circadian dose without fully sitting up and without turning a light on. They should then be able to go back to sleep. This should all take less than 30 seconds. Some thyroid patients with weak adrenals find that they need to urinate during the night, and when they wake up to take the circadian dose, a visit to the bathroom may be necessary. Ideally, this visit should also be done with the light off so that the thyroid patient has the best chance of going back to sleep.

THE CIRCADIAN T3 METHOD STEP BY STEP

CT3M is applied in this way:

1. Symptoms, signs and cortisol test results (ideally a twenty-four hour adrenal saliva test result) are reviewed. These results can be used to determine if CT3M should be applied.

2. An alarm clock, mobile phone alarm, or some other alarm will be needed, and should be set to the time that the circadian dose is to be taken.

3. **Thyroid patients have found that a starting dose of 10 micrograms, taken at one and a half hours before getting up, is an effective way to start CT3M.** For someone who gets up at 8:00 am, this would mean taking a 10 microgram circadian dose of T3 (or one grain of NDT) medication, at approximately 6:30 am. Some thyroid patients who are very sensitive to thyroid medication begin at only 5 micrograms of T3 containing medication, and occasionally even less than this.

4. **Then, wait for a few days, or even a week.** Evaluate the response. This means attempting to see if there has been any positive effect from the circadian dose. This may be an improvement in one or more symptoms or one or more signs (like body temperature or blood pressure). It may also be a general feeling of improved well-being and energy level. It may take a few days to see any response to the circadian dose. Typically, improvements might be a slightly higher body temperature in the morning or later in the day, or a higher blood pressure (if it was low to begin with). Improved symptoms might include better energy levels or simply feeling less ill. Some people respond immediately, and in others the response takes a few days, or a week or more, to occur.

5. **If there has been no noticeable positive response to the starting circadian dose then it can be increased in steps of 2.5 micrograms or 5 micrograms** until some positive response is seen in symptoms and signs. For NDT this would mean an increase of 1/4-1/2 grain.

6. Ideally, at least a week should be present between dosage changes, but a minimum of two to three days needs to be allowed. The periods between dosage changes are necessary in order to allow time for changes in adrenal performance, and to assess a new circadian dose properly. It is hard to be prescriptive about how long to wait because some dosage changes take time to come to fruition. Particular attention should be paid to blood pressure, as improved adrenal function can raise blood pressure. It is important to be patient at this stage, because cortisol levels can take several weeks to fully adjust, even though some benefits may be detectable within days. Cortisol levels may not stabilise for several weeks after a circadian dose change.

7. **If the thyroid patient is using adrenal glandulars or adrenal steroids, then these should not be used until at least four hours (ideally longer) after the circadian dose of T3 containing medication has been taken.** This is to avoid the adrenal steroid medication suppressing the natural production of adrenal hormones. As with all things, there may be exceptions to this if the patient's doctor believes that the thyroid patient cannot function without some adrenal steroid earlier than this.

8. A positive response to the circadian dose is often achieved with 10, 12.5 or 15 micrograms of T3 containing medication. **The response only needs to be detectable** - it does not need to provide a significant improvement in symptoms. There needs to be some response so that when the circadian dose timing is adjusted it can be assessed using symptoms and signs. If the circadian dose is too large at this stage, then moving it earlier may elicit too great a response from the adrenal glands. Hence 10, 12.5 or 15 micrograms are typical levels after this first adjustment in circadian dose size (although some thyroid patients do need more, and a few need even less).

9. **Once some positive response of the circadian dose is experienced, then the timing of the circadian dose is adjusted by taking it half an hour earlier.** The response in symptoms and signs is monitored once more. The change should typically be held for around a week before further adjustments should they be necessary.

10. **The timing of the circadian dose should not need to be earlier than four hours prior to getting up, which with an 8:00 am get-up time would be 4:00 am.** I do know of people who have moved the circadian dose to four and a half hours before getting up, and they believe that this is more beneficial to them.

11. Even a change of half an hour can alter cortisol levels, so allowing time to evaluate each change is important. The goal of this stage of timing adjustment is to locate the most effective time to take the circadian dose for the individual thyroid patient (the 'sweet spot' for the circadian dose timing). Everyone is different, and some thyroid patients do well with a circadian dose taken only 1.5 hours before get-up time. Others need much earlier times, such as 2, 3 or 4 hours before rising in the morning.

12. **After adjusting and determining the most effective time to take the circadian dose, the circadian dose size may be fine-tuned.** This would only be done if it were believed that the thyroid patient's adrenal performance was still under par. During this dose size adjustment stage, the circadian dose could be increased by 2.5 or 5 micrograms of T3, or 1/4-1/2 grain of NDT. The response should be monitored and then the dose size may be adjusted further if necessary.

13. If the adrenal response was too great, the size of the circadian dose could be decreased or the timing could be moved forward (later in time) by half an hour. In some circumstances, where there appears to be a profound effect due to a 30-minute change in circadian dose timing, some thyroid patients have adopted timing changes of 10 or 15 minutes and found this to be helpful. This is not a common need, but it is something to keep in mind.

14. If there is confusion over what is going on at any time, the process can be reset. For instance, by reducing the circadian dose to 10 micrograms of T3 containing medication and taking it at one and half hours before getting up. Or simply reverting back to a circadian dose and a timing that appeared to be more stable. The process can then be repeated.

15. The typical range of T3 required for the circadian dose to successfully apply CT3M is between 10 and 30 micrograms, with 15 to 25 micrograms being more typical. If NDT were being used then, this would commonly be between one grain (about 60 mg of NDT) and two and a half grains (about 150 mg of NDT).

16. For thyroid patients using natural desiccated thyroid, or any hard tablet based NDT to provide the T3, then it should be chewed up well before swallowing to enable fast absorption.

17. If necessary, timing and possibly size adjustments to all other T3 or NDT daytime doses may be needed as a result of the impact of improved adrenal performance caused by the circadian dose.

18. CT3M often raises adrenal hormones and sex hormones. Women have reported higher oestrogen levels, and increased testosterone has been measured in men. As CT3M is applied, the improved adrenal output can radically boost the action of daytime T3 doses or NDT doses. As a result of this 'super-charging' of daytime thyroid medication, any daytime

doses may need fine-tuning (often reduction) to work more effectively with the circadian dose.

19. Ideally, when applying CT3M, the daytime T3 or NDT doses will be maintained at low enough sizes to avoid problems. This may mean reducing the daytime doses in order to remain slightly under-medicated during the day whilst the circadian dose is being titrated. If this is not done, then there is a risk of excessive adrenal hormones or sex hormones being produced due to too high a level of daytime thyroid medication.

20. It is also important to be aware that if the daytime doses of thyroid medication are far too low then this is enough to seriously undermine adrenal performance. This is covered within Chapter 8 of this book.

21. At various points during this process, it may be important to gather more laboratory test data. The twenty-four hour adrenal saliva test may need to be repeated at intervals to provide concrete evidence of the effect of CT3M and to assess actual cortisol levels. A sex hormone panel may also be valuable. It is very important to actually assess cortisol levels through a laboratory test. This is to avoid attempting to guess whether the cortisol output is adequate or not, simply based on symptoms alone. Symptomatic assessment of cortisol levels can be very misleading. If aldosterone had also been a concern, then this would need testing. A sex hormone panel may also be valuable.

22. When the circadian dose size and timing are thought to be almost ideal, then symptoms and signs may be used to determine if further fine-tuning of the circadian dose, or of the daytime doses, is required.

The above process is repeated until a good and stable response is obtained. This can take some time, as the adrenal glands need time to recover. If adjusting the circadian dose is not able to correct adrenal function, then the thyroid patient and their doctor might need to consider the use of some form of adrenal support. Alternatively, they may need to investigate other health issues that may be disrupting CT3M (see Chapter 8).

REPEATING THE TWENTY-FOUR HOUR ADRENAL SALIVA TEST

As part of the process of determining if CT3M is relevant, many thyroid patients will have sensibly undertaken a twenty-four hour adrenal saliva test. Once the CT3M process is being used, it is important to repeat this test from time-to-time. It can often be extremely difficult to determine if cortisol is low or high (without this test), as both of these situations can adversely affect thyroid hormone action. Consequently, when there has been slow progress, or the thyroid patient and their doctor are not sure what is actually happening, then a repeat of the twenty-four hour adrenal saliva test is advisable. Getting the real data regarding the profile of free/biologically active cortisol in the body over the day can be immensely helpful. If progress is very good, the need to repeat this test will not be so great and the thyroid patient and their doctor may be able to wait for a while to retest this.

ADDITIONAL OPTIONS

For those thyroid patients who find that after several months of applying CT3M they need a little more help with adrenal function, there are many avenues that can be investigated.

Chapter 8 discusses the many situations or conditions that can adversely affect thyroid hormone action and CT3M. Each of these areas could be investigated. In particular, some thyroid patients do find value in combining LDN use with CT3M (some even taking the LDN at the same time as the circadian dose), as LDN appears to help improve cortisol for some patients. This should of course be discussed with the patient's own doctor. See Chapter 20 for more information about LDN.

In Chapter 20, I will discuss the optional use of a small bedtime dose of thyroid medication, which has been found to be of benefit to some thyroid patients.

Chapter 12

Exceptions to The Basic CT3M Process

Most processes or methods need to be modified from time to time. CT3M is no exception. The majority of thyroid patients that use CT3M use it according to the process that I have outlined in Chapter 11. However, occasionally someone may have unique requirements that dictate some change to the basic CT3M, or a more radical change to the process.

It is not possible to comprehensively define all the possible ways in which CT3M might need to be modified. I can guarantee that in the future, a thyroid patient will come forward with some specific reason dictating something novel that I have not listed here, nor even considered. However, I will attempt to mention the ways that a small number of thyroid patients have needed to break the basic CT3M process.

LOW STARTING DOSES (UNDER 10-MICROGRAM DOSES OF T3)

In a small number of cases, the typical starting dose of around 10 micrograms of T3, or 1 grain of NDT, has been found to be too much for some thyroid patients to cope with. There appear to be two reasons why some people react in this way:

1. A few thyroid patients only appear to need a tiny amount of T3 or NDT to realise the benefit of CT3M. In this case, the starting dose of T3-containing medication of 10 micrograms produces either symptoms of over-stimulation by thyroid hormone, or excess cortisol or other adrenal hormones. Symptoms alone can often suggest what is happening, but laboratory testing of adrenal hormones may also suggest that there is a problem. As I've mentioned before, the twenty-four hour adrenal saliva test can be an invaluable tool in confirming that the circadian dose has been too powerful.

2. The second reason why this can occasionally occur is when the thyroid patient's adrenal glands cannot immediately respond to even a 10-microgram circadian dose of T3, or 1 grain of NDT. In this case, the thyroid medication may place more demand than the adrenal glands can support. A lack of adrenal gland response can cause a rise in adrenaline that may be mistaken for sensitivity to thyroid medication. (see Chapter 7 where this is discussed).

One technique to explore in either of these situations is to try circadian doses as low as 5 or 7.5 micrograms of T3, or the equivalent of NDT. In some extremely rare cases, the thyroid patient may find that only a circadian dose as low as 2.5 micrograms can be tolerated to begin with.

Some thyroid patients that have very low cortisol may respond to CT3M with symptoms that appear to suggest elevated adrenaline, e.g. a high heart rate when trying to raise thyroid hormone (see Chapter 7 for more details). In these cases, taking a small circadian dose at the start of the main cortisol production window (4 hours before getting up) can be helpful. In a few cases, a thyroid patient who uses a low circadian dose at 4 hours before getting up can find that this is tolerated well. This approach provides less T3 stimulation through the entire period of high adrenal activity. Once the adrenals perform better, then this dose may be raised and the timing can be adjusted at a later date. No process can cope with every eventuality, and occasionally techniques like this might be needed in special cases.

Whatever reason is responsible for the issues, usually low doses will only need to be sustained for a short time. This should only be until a better response is achieved, or the underlying reason for any poor response to CT3M is discovered and corrected. For a very small number of people, a very low circadian dose will be all that they ever need. I know of one lady who has been very successful for a long time now with only a 6.25-microgram circadian dose.

Since the use of very small circadian doses is rarely of help to the majority of thyroid patients, the CT3M process recommends starting with a circadian dose of 10 micrograms, or 1 grain NDT. I still feel that this is an excellent starting point in general.

HIGH CIRCADIAN DOSES (ABOVE 25-30 MICROGRAMS OF T3)

CT3M rarely requires circadian doses above 25 or 30 micrograms of T3 (approximately 3 grains of NDT). However, very occasionally a thyroid patient may require a circadian dose that is much higher. The CT3M process allows for this possibility, and if the rare thyroid patient finds that CT3M only works with a higher circadian dose, then this is technically within the bounds of the process.

The majority of thyroid patients using CT3M will find that a circadian dose that contains between 10 and 25 micrograms of T3 (or the equivalent of NDT - 1 grain to 2.5 grains of NDT), will be the optimal level of circadian dose required.

CIRCADIAN DOSES LATER THAN 1.5 HOURS BEFORE GETTING UP

CT3M is explicit about the circadian dose being taken at least 1.5 hours before the thyroid patient gets up out of bed in the morning. This is a good guideline, and works in the vast majority of cases. At the time of writing this book, CT3M has been used by vast numbers of thyroid patients all over the world for around eighteen months. During that time a tiny number of people have found that taking the circadian dose at 1.5 hours before getting up is too effective, in that it may produce far too much response from the adrenal glands and drive cortisol in the morning to beyond the ideal level.

If a thyroid patient and their doctor discover that the adrenal response is too great, then a later time for the circadian dose can be considered, e.g. 1 hour before the thyroid patient gets up. This is rare, and should not be considered unless there is clear evidence that it is required.

One problem to be aware of is that in a few cases of implementing CT3M, sex hormones like estradiol and testosterone may also rise. There appear to be some individuals for whom these hormones can become excessive with certain circadian dose timings (often in the 1.5 - 2.5 hour before getting up region). In this particular case, moving the circadian dose later may correct the sex hormone rise, but it may not be ideal for adrenal hormones like cortisol. In this case, the patient and their own doctor may wish to consider moving the circadian dose earlier in time (2.5 - 4 hours before the patient gets up). This is in order to avoid over-stimulation of sex hormones and still gain a good improvement in adrenal steroids.

CIRCADIAN DOSES EARLIER THAN 4 HOURS BEFORE GETTING UP

Very occasionally, a circadian dose taken more than 4 hours before the thyroid patient gets up may effective. If a thyroid patient has seen improvements in moving the circadian dose to an earlier time but is still not totally well, then occasionally it may make some sense to take the circadian dose slightly earlier than 4 hours before getting up. The decision to do this would depend on whether all other ideas for improvement have been exhausted, because in the majority of cases this will not help. Even in this case, I would not recommend taking the circadian dose earlier than 4.5 or 5 hours before the thyroid patient rises, as the endocrinology of the circadian pattern of cortisol production does not appear to support this.

TIME ADJUSTMENTS SMALLER THAN 30 MINUTES

The CT3M process describes adjusting the time of the circadian dose in 30-minute increments. I can state that some thyroid patients have noticed changes in adrenal performance when using only 10 - 15 minute changes to the circadian dose timing. Whilst this may not apply to everyone, it may be worth considering during the fine-tuning process, particularly if someone appears very sensitive to time changes.

A COMBINED NDT/T3 OR T4 CIRCADIAN DOSE

Both the *Recovering with T3* book (and Chapter 5 of this book), describe the use of T3 only or NDT only medication options for the circadian dose. A few thyroid patients have broken this process with some success.

A few thyroid patients have combined NDT and T3 for the circadian dose. It is not common at all. However, when a thyroid patient has combined NDT and T3, or T4 and T3 in the circadian dose, it has invariably been due to the need to raise FT3 and lower reverse T3. This may have come about as a result of thyroid blood tests that have shown the levels of both FT3 and reverse T3. Finding an appropriate balance of NDT and T3 combined doses can involve a substantial amount of trial and error, and is not something to be taken on lightly - there would need to be an extremely good reason to venture down this route. However, I do know of a few people who have found this to be helpful.

I am also aware of one thyroid patient who has used a circadian dose of levothyroxine (synthetic T4). They say that this has really improved their adrenal function. For this to have had any benefit at all, I would argue that the thyroid patient must have had excellent conversion of T4 to T3. It is not something that should be considered as a serious option by thyroid patients and their doctors; unless, that is, the thyroid patient has excellent high end of the reference range FT3 levels. Even then I would not expect this to aid adrenal function for most people. I include this here for completeness, but this is the only instance I know of.

CONTNUATION OF ADRENAL GLANDULARS OR STEROIDS ALONGSIDE CT3M

The goal of CT3M is to support the adrenal glands and allow them to function normally again, with healthy levels of cortisol and other adrenal hormones being produced. This is best done with no adrenal glandulars or adrenal steroids (such as hydrocortisone) being used. Since CT3M has been introduced, thyroid patients and their doctors have learned how best to wean any existing adrenal glandular products or adrenal steroids as CT3M begins to be applied. The process for weaning adrenal steroids is covered in Chapter 19.

In a very small number of cases, the thyroid patient and their doctor may decide that it is too dangerous to the health of the thyroid patient for any adrenal steroids to be weaned completely, or even partly. This decision is taken usually because the thyroid patient is suspected of having the early stages of Addison's disease or some level of hypopituitarism. In these cases, to remove the exogenous adrenal steroids would be a mistake, even though some small reduction in them might be tolerated.

CT3M is generally not used in cases of Addison's disease or hypopituitarism. However, in cases where these conditions are not extreme, CT3M may still be of help. I know of a handful of cases where CT3M has proved to be of benefit even though the thyroid patients have remained on some level of adrenal steroids. The number of these situations is very small, but again it is worth mentioning here to illustrate that processes like CT3M should not be followed slavishly in every single case. One example of success with this approach may be found in Chapter 22 (see 'Francis's Story').

Chapter 13

Circadian Dose Timing and Size Adjustments

Adjustment to both the timing and size of the circadian dose are necessary.

A change to the time the circadian dose is taken provides a gentle change of FT3 level to the adrenal glands. A later (i.e. closer to getting up time) T3 dose ensures slightly less FT3 arrives inside the adrenal cells over the entire period when they are producing early morning cortisol. This often produces a lower response from the adrenal glands. An earlier T3 dose allows slightly more FT3 within the adrenal cells, and may produce a larger response.

A change to the size of the circadian dose can produce very large effects. Even small increases of 2.5 micrograms of T3 containing medication can substantially increase FT3 levels in the cells.

Ideally, just sufficient T3 containing medication will be used, but it will be taken early enough in the cycle of adrenal hormone production that it will fully support the adrenal glands.

CIRCADIAN DOSE TIMING ADJUSTMENT

As covered in Chapter 11, CT3M begins by finding the smallest circadian dose size that has some positive effect on symptoms or signs, and which is taken at one and a half hours before getting up. This initial circadian dose does not need to fully resolve symptoms - only to result in some **detectable benefit**.

Once the initial circadian dose is large enough to produce some noticeable effect (no matter how minor), then time adjustment to the circadian dose may provide a smoother change in adrenal function. **Adjusting the time of the circadian dose is the fine-tuning dial on the adrenal glands in CT3M.** Hence it is better to find the smallest possible circadian dose that appears to have some positive effect at one and a half hours before getting up, and then adjust the time of the dose to find the optimal time to take it. Only once the optimal time is found should the circadian dose be increased to discover the best dose size. This 'optimal time' may also need to be fine-tuned at some point once again.

It is worth noting that occasionally uncomfortable symptoms may be experienced with intermediate timings of a circadian dose. Only when the circadian dose is ideally timed for a thyroid patient might they feel an improvement.

CIRCADIAN DOSE SIZE ADJUSTMENT

If the circadian dose is increased too much when taken at one and a half hours before getting up, it can become far too potent for the adrenal glands when the circadian dose is moved back to an earlier time. This may cause symptoms associated with high cortisol, or over-stress the adrenal glands and cause symptoms of even lower cortisol than the thyroid patient began with. Consequently, thyroid patients have found that using a circadian dose of 10, 12.5 or 15 micrograms at one and half hours before getting up is often a good starting point before adjusting the circadian dose in time.

If the initial circadian dose size is only slightly effective, then titrating it back in time is an ideal way to proceed. The initial circadian dose size does not need to resolve all symptoms, or even any symptoms; it only needs to be seen to have some positive effect. Hence only a small increase from a starting circadian dose of 10 micrograms of T3 containing medication may be necessary. Some sensitive thyroid patients may need to begin with an even lower dose of T3 medication than 10 micrograms.

In the *Recovering with T3* book, I describe how I see T3 medication behaving as though it is a wave[RWT3 1]:

"For each divided dose of T3, I discovered that there was definitely a 'threshold level' that had to be exceeded before any real benefit was experienced from the hormone. As I increased the dose beyond this threshold level then the effects were greater. If I exceeded the threshold too much then I experienced symptoms of tissue over-stimulation. My threshold level tended to be lower as the day progressed. So, later in the day I required lower doses of T3 to achieve the same effect. This perception may be due in part to some cumulative effect of the previous doses of T3 but the interaction with other hormones, which reduce in level during the day, may also be relevant.

I often use a specific analogy to describe to other people how T3 appears to behave:
Imagine a sandy beach, which is sheltered from the sea by large rocks. Only a wave that is large and powerful enough is capable of striking the rocks and sending a spray of seawater over them to drench the sand beyond."

If I apply this concept to CT3M, then it can be seen that as the circadian dose is increased, the size of the *wave of T3* increases, and significantly more FT3 becomes available to the adrenals. This is not subtle or manageable. It should be possible to understand that adjusting the size of a circadian dose by even 2.5 micrograms can produce a profoundly different effect. **Consequently, adjusting the size of the circadian dose may be viewed as the rough-tuning dial on our adrenal glands in CT3M.**

THERE IS NO OPTIMAL TIME AND SIZE OF CIRCADIAN DOSE - EVERYONE IS DIFFERENT

The optimal time to take the circadian dose varies a great deal between thyroid patients. In general, those thyroid patients with very low cortisol appear to do better when the circadian dose is taken earlier in the main cortisol production window, perhaps in the 2.5 to 4 hours before getting-up region. For those thyroid patients that have only moderately low cortisol, they will often find that a time of 1.5 to 2.5 hours before getting up is adequate. If they move the circadian dose earlier than this, they may feel worse due to far too high an effect on the adrenal glands.

Once the ideal time has been found to take the circadian dose, then the circadian dose size may be increased further if necessary. After this, further fine-tuning of both time and size of the circadian dose may be performed as required based on symptoms and signs.

It should be obvious from the above that both the time adjustment *and* the circadian dose size adjustment are necessary. This is in order to fine tune CT3M, and optimally support the adrenal glands for those thyroid patients with partial adrenal insufficiency. This should explain why most thyroid patients should not just begin CT3M with a circadian dose taken 4 hours before they get up in the morning (which is something I have been asked about from time to time by people who desire to simplify the process).

In addition to the above, it is now clear that some people may need to take their circadian dose slightly closer to their get-up (i.e. rising) time than the 1.5 hours suggested within the basic process. Although, the closer that this becomes to getting up, the greater the risk that the individual will not be able to return to sleep. I now know of a few people who do well with a circadian dose taken 1 hour before they get up. In terms of the circadian dose size itself, there are a few people who only need extremely small doses of T3 in the order of 5 micrograms (around ½ grain NDT), and some that require more than 25 micrograms. These types of timing and dose sizes for the circadian dose are relatively unusual, but they do happen.

IS THERE A 'SWEET SPOT' FOR CIRCADIAN DOSE TIMING?

I've heard this question many times. I do not believe that there is a permanent ideal timing or dose size for a circadian dose. When a thyroid patient has partial adrenal insufficiency, it should be possible to apply CT3M and find a workable dose time and size. These may both change over time as the adrenals improve.

As I've already mentioned, generally speaking, an earlier circadian dose time will provide a better, more powerful response from the adrenal glands. This is the best working assumption to make for most thyroid patients. Some thyroid patients find that they do better with circadian dose times that are later, or in the middle of, the main cortisol production window. There is no great surprise in this. Finding the best time to take the circadian dose is all that is important.

One of the most common mistakes is finding a time for the circadian dose that appears to have some benefit, and then never moving it back earlier in time. I have spoken to thyroid patients who have only explored circadian dose timings in the 1.5 to 2.5 hours range before getting up. This can often completely ignore the potential for greater improvement when the circadian dose is taken earlier in time - perhaps in the 2.5 to 4 hour range before getting up. Making a timing adjustment may also require a dose size adjustment (lower or higher).

A good example of this was provided to me in writing by a thyroid patient, who wrote:

"I started CT3M with a very small dose at about 1½ hours before normal waking time, but always became nauseous within a few minutes – and it lasted for several hours after waking. However, I persisted because adrenal supplements made me feel "wired" once I started CT3M, so I knew it must be working. This nausea continued even when I moved back to 2 hours and then 2½ hours. It was ONLY when I then jumped to 3½ and then 4 hours before waking time that this nausea stopped. Yes, I do have fairly serious adrenal issues.

You (me in *Recovering with T3*) do state that those with more serious adrenal issues will need to take the circadian dose 3-4 hours before getting up, but what I would like is to see a warning that - for such people - there may be nausea when working backwards to the 3-4 hour time. This might encourage some people to work more quickly backwards as I did. I am wondering how many just gave up, instead? Those of us with serious adrenal issues need CT3M the most, and there is not really any other way to rebuild the adrenal glands (except perhaps the herbal tincture rhodioloa rosea). Oh yes, throughout 20 years all of my standard lab tests showed normal!

Once again, thank you for your book and for inventing CT3M (brilliant!). I relished your careful logic throughout. When I first read your book, I thought you were too careful and too pedantic in your approach to T3. After a couple of disastrous initial weeks, I re-read your book and appreciated every millimetre of your caution. I clearly needed to get the circadian dose back to between three and four hours before getting up, but had issues with the intervening times that the circadian dose was taken. This is a good reminder that in the case of quite severe partial adrenal insufficiency, that persisting with CT3M can be very beneficial, and that sometimes moving the circadian dose more quickly can be advantageous."

I thought that the above observations were immensely insightful and relevant to many people. However, I would not like to see this as a general rule that all thyroid patients with severe partial adrenal insufficiency should take their circadian dose at 3-4 hours before getting up. It does serve as a reminder though, that in some cases changing the dose timing more quickly may be helpful. It is also a reminder that just because intervening dose timings are not effective does not mean that an earlier time of 3-4 hours before getting up won't be highly effective.

Whatever time or dose size is found that works for CT3M, then over time these may need to be adjusted as the adrenals and the health of the thyroid patient improves.

DAYTIME DOSING OF THYROID MEDICATION

The daytime doses of thyroid medication may be too high or too low as CT3M is applied. In addition, some women have reported higher oestrogen or testosterone levels, and increased testosterone has been measured in men.

As CT3M is applied, improved adrenal output can radically boost the action of daytime T3 doses or NDT doses. As a result of this 'super-charging' of daytime thyroid medication, any daytime doses may need fine-tuning (often reduction) to work more effectively with the circadian dose. Ideally, when applying CT3M, the daytime T3 doses or NDT doses will be maintained at low enough sizes to avoid problems. This may mean reducing the daytime doses in order to remain slightly under-medicated during the day whilst the circadian dose is being titrated. If this is not done, there is a risk of excessive adrenal or sex hormones being produced due to too high a level of daytime thyroid medication.

If the daytime doses of thyroid medication are too low, then CT3M alone may not be sufficient to maintain an improved level of adrenal performance. The adrenal glands also need T3 thyroid hormone during the day. If they are starved of enough T3 during the day, even an optimal circadian dose will not enable them to recover the next morning.

Consequently, a subtle balance is needed in daytime thyroid medication. Daytime thyroid doses of T3 or NDT should not be so large as to risk becoming over-stimulatory, but equally they should not be so low that they prevent the recovery of the adrenal glands.

ADJUSTMENTS TO THE TIMING AND SIZE OF CIRCADIAN DOSE

In the CT3M process described within Chapter 11 of this book, I suggest that time changes should be in 30-minute steps, and that the dose size adjustment should be between 2.5 and 5 micrograms of T3 (or the equivalent of NDT). This is typical, and usually works quite well. These are certainly the right order of changes to be making during the early stages of applying CT3M.

Eventually, there may come a point when fine-tuning is required. At this stage, I would definitely say that 2.5 microgram changes in T3 doses (around one quarter of a grain of NDT), should be adopted, as the largest amount of change to consider. Larger changes may work, but the change may be too big and produce results that appear worse, thereby running the risk of passing the ideal dosage.

A small number of thyroid patients may also benefit from smaller changes in circadian dose time during fine-tuning e.g. 15 minute changes may benefit some people who appear sensitive to subtle time changes in the circadian dose.

Chapter 14

Get Up Versus Wake Up Time

The natural circadian rhythm of cortisol production should ensure that the highest volume of cortisol is produced during the last four hours of sleep. I describe this critical four-hour period as the *main cortisol production window.* [RWT3 1]

Thyroid patients often ask questions about the main cortisol production window. Typical questions include:

- Do I use the time I wake up, or when I get out of bed, as the end of the main cortisol production window?
- When is the end of this critical four hours?
- What if someone wakes up several times before getting up?
- What if someone doesn't go back to sleep after taking the circadian dose?

The CT3M process makes the simple assumption that the end of the main cortisol production window is when the thyroid patient <u>gets up out of bed</u> in the morning. The reason for this assumption is simple - there is no way to be certain of exactly how the individual's sleep pattern is affecting the natural cortisol production rhythm. Some assumption has to be used as a starting point, and then trial and error will determine the ideal circadian dose and timing. The CT3M process will enable a range of circadian dose times to be explored. This simplistic approach has been found to be reasonably effective.

DIFFICULTIES GOING BACK TO SLEEP AFTER THE CIRCADIAN DOSE

Some thyroid patients have complained they have difficulty sleeping once they have turned off their alarm and taken their circadian dose. If the circadian dose is taken quickly, with no need to turn a light on, then going back to sleep should not be an issue for most thyroid patients (even a short trip to the bathroom in darkness should not be a real issue for most people).

However, for a few, the actual act of taking a circadian dose is disruptive to their sleep, and they genuinely struggle to sleep again afterwards. This disruption to sleep often resolves once CT3M has been applied and the circadian dose has been fine-tuned. This is because poor quality of sleep is frequently linked to high or low cortisol levels. The process of using CT3M is designed to improve the performance of the adrenal glands, which may produce a better sleeping pattern and deeper and more refreshing sleep.

A very small number of people may find that a disrupted sleep pattern is something that they cannot tolerate, such is the impact of this on their lives. In these rare cases, it may be advisable to give up on attempting to use CT3M, and instead resort to other means of correcting partial adrenal insufficiency.

Chapter 15

Handling Getting Up Time, Time Zone or Other Changes

Once a circadian dose has been established that appears to be working effectively, inevitably there will be some normal variation in the time that a thyroid patient gets up out of bed in the morning. I am frequently asked whether the timing of the circadian dose should be altered where variations to a patient's standard schedule occurs.

The reasons for these variations are many, but might include:

- Getting up for work at a fixed time during the week, but at a later time at the weekends.
- Getting up at a fixed time during the week to get children off to school, or to support a partner preparing for work, and then changing this schedule at the weekend.
- A work schedule that occasionally demands a very early or late start to the day.
- Occasional travel for work or a holiday, involving entering a different time zone - perhaps with a several hour time difference.
- Shift work in cycles of a week (or several weeks) on one shift, and then adjusting to a different shift. This is particularly hard on the adrenal glands and the endocrine system.
- Erratic patterns of waking and sleeping, which may result for many reasons. However, in some cases the pattern may not be consistent each day. In the worst case, it may involve sleeping for a few hours during the day or in the night when it is possible to do so.

As you read down the above bulleted list, the exceptions and variations to a fairly standard and healthy sleep pattern become more severe. The last item on the list describes a relatively uncommon situation, but one that is very extreme. The first item on the list is very typical for many thyroid patients who work.

A TYPICAL 5-DAY SLEEP / GET-UP PATTERN WITH 2 DAYS DIFFERENT

The first three items on the list describe the getting-up pattern for the majority of thyroid patients. Each of these scenarios is essentially the same as the others.

For a thyroid patient who is applying CT3M, then I would say that if they have the same get-up time for 4 or 5 days of the week, then this get-up time should be assumed to be the end of the main cortisol production window. In other words, no adjustment should be made to the timing of the circadian dose for the non-standard 2 or 3 days of the week.

The reason for this is that the adrenals and HPA axis take some time to adjust when a change in get-up time occurs. Sleeping later at the weekend will make such little difference to the adrenals for most people that the circadian dose timing should just continue to be the same time for all 7 days of the week. This is the best assumption for those that only have 2 or 3 days a week where there is a variation in schedule. If a thyroid patient discovers that they are particularly sensitive, and some difference is felt, then they may choose to make their own adjustment on the exception days - the majority of patients will not need to do this.

TIME ZONE OR SHIFT WORK CHANGES

Significant time zone changes and shift work may be an entirely more problematic issue. If someone spends only a very short amount of time on a totally different sleep/wake cycle, then they may be able to keep taking their thyroid medication (including the circadian dose) at exactly the same times they were previously doing. For this to work however, the shift change or time in the new time zone would have to be of the order of a few days only.

For time zone or shift changes that involve the person staying on the new time zone or shift for many days (or a week or more), then the circadian dose timing will need to be adjusted to fit in with the new sleep/wake pattern. Even if this adjustment is made, the adrenals and HPA axis may take some time to adjust. It can take weeks for changes to be completely made in the body to a new time zone or a new shift. This is why shift work is so hard on the body - the endocrine system is in permanent catch-up mode. However, there would be no choice but to make the timing change to the circadian dose and move it to about the same time before the new get-up time as it was in the previous sleep/wake cycle. After this initial change, some further fine-tuning may also be necessary. Unfortunately, the new shift or time zone may not be in operation for weeks and may revert back to the old one, causing the thyroid patient to have to re-adjust once more. If this is for the purpose of a holiday, then it may be coped with relatively easily. But if it is a regular occurrence due to work needs, then it can be very hard to cope with indeed. Some people may find that this disruption due to shift work, or regular significant time zone changes, makes it very difficult to obtain the types of results that they want to see from CT3M.

VERY ERRATIC SLEEP WAKE CYCLES

I'll now cover the last category of people who have very erratic patterns of sleep and wake, which are far more problematic to implementing CT3M successfully.

I mean no criticism in any of this as often such people have fallen into this situation through various life events, or jobs that have necessitated a less than typical pattern of sleep or extremely poor adrenal function. Let me start by talking about the link between some hormones and sleep/wake or night/day. Early human beings went to sleep after it was dark and rose in the morning when it was light. Our bodies are designed for this. Many hormones are linked to the night/day cycle. These hormones include growth hormone, thyroid hormones and sex hormones. Cortisol is slightly different, being linked to our sleep/wake cycle so that we are ready for action when we do wake up.

All the hormones are designed to work together. Ideally, cortisol production will occur in the last four hours of sleep and be in synchronisation with other hormones to gain the optimal effect. Consequently, it is not surprising that some thyroid patients have found that CT3M works more effectively when they adapt their sleep wake times to a more natural timing.

For those with a very erratic pattern of sleeping and waking, this change may be something that they find very difficult to do. However, for someone with a very poor sleep/wake cycle, adjusting this cycle and trying to make it more typical may be the only way to be able to apply CT3M and achieve any benefit from it.

In our modern world, some people go to bed and get up in the morning out of synchronisation with the night/day cycle. There are many people who rise early in the morning, say at 6:00 am, before it is fully light. There are others who only rise at 11:00am or noon. For these people, the hormones that are linked to the night/day cycle will be out of synchronisation with cortisol production. In the majority of cases this may not matter greatly. But for some thyroid patients with adrenal issues who are using CT3M, this may be a problem. For example, if a thyroid patient using CT3M takes their circadian dose at 9:00 am and gets out of bed at noon, they may fare better getting up at 9:00 am and taking the circadian dose at 6:00 am. Any change such as this should be done slowly in 30 to 60 minute steps over time.

For someone who snoozes for only a hour or so at a time, and does so at random times over 24 hours, then trying to re-establish a sleep/wake cycle by going to bed before midnight and rising in the morning may be exceptionally difficult. However, it may be the only way to get any value from CT3M. Perhaps CT3M may not be something that can be considered. I am clearly not making this a recommendation as part of the protocol for using CT3M, but our bodies do work in this way, and some thyroid patients may wish to consider sleep/wake cycle changes as part of an overall health improvement programme. The majority of thyroid patients are not likely to have to consider this, as their adrenals will improve perfectly well without any change to the timing of when they sleep or wake. This is simply a note for those few that may continue to have problems and who have more unusual sleep patterns.

CLOCK ADJUSTMENTS TWICE PER YEAR

In Chapter 18 of *Recovering with T3* I describe how to adjust the circadian dose when a national clock change for summer or wintertime occurs.

Here is the text that appears in *Recovering with T3*:

"In the UK all of our clocks are adjusted twice per year. In the spring we move them forward by an hour to adopt British Summer Time (BST). In the autumn, at the end of BST we adjust them back by an hour to Greenwich Mean Time (GMT). After a clock adjustment, I discovered that my body clock wasn't able to change overnight with the clock change. Therefore, at the end of BST (in the autumn) I move the timing of my first dose of T3 by between half an hour and one hour earlier. At the start of BST (in the spring) I do the opposite and move the timing of my first dose of T3 later by half an hour to one hour. Anyone who is affected by seasonal clock changes might need to consider this. This can be especially critical for someone using the Circadian T3 Method."

The above shows how the circadian dose is adjusted when a national clock change occurs. If the clock change moves the time later by one hour, then the alarm clock for the circadian dose should be moved later by 30 to 60 minutes. If the clock change moves the time earlier by one hour, then the circadian dose need to be moved earlier by 30 to 60 minutes.

Chapter 16

Symptoms and Signs

This chapter provides an overview of symptoms and signs that thyroid patients and their doctors may find useful to monitor whilst assessing the progress of CT3M. The guidelines in this chapter are a starting point, and will not cover all cases and all patients' needs.

For more information on using symptoms and signs, the reader should review *Recovering with T3*, [RWT3 1] which includes the following two extracts within Chapter 21:

"Doctors use the terms 'symptoms' and 'signs' in a very specific way. A symptom is something that the patient complains about or feels. A sign is a specific observation or measurement that has a more objective value and that someone else can observe or measure. One example is body temperature. If I complained that I was feeling cold and my body temperature reading was below normal, then the sign would be the temperature measurement and the symptom would be my sensitivity to cold."

"Symptoms and signs provide vital clues that can be used to assess whether a dosage change has been effective or detrimental. They have enabled me to decide whether I have needed more T3 in any given dose, whether the dose has been correct, or whether it has been too high and has led to any risk from tissue over-stimulation. Symptoms and signs are also important in the assessment of the timing of divided doses. I was able to determine when the positive effects of each T3 divided dose were declining and only take another divided dose when absolutely necessary."

GENERAL OBSERVATIONS

Both high and low cortisol can cause thyroid hormones to be rendered less effective. High cortisol can block the effect of thyroid hormone; low cortisol can reduce the flow of glucose from the bloodstream to the cells and also make thyroid hormone less effective (due to the adverse effect on ATP production). Consequently, it is important to be aware when using CT3M, that it is very easy to be confused as to whether cortisol levels are high or low.

It is also important to remember that if the thyroid patient has serious partial adrenal insufficiency, and the circadian dose is increased or moved earlier, then this can cause too much strain on the adrenals. Hence, rather than getting an improvement, you can see a worsening of symptoms and signs. There can be a need for considerable trial and error, and careful thinking at times.

Another valuable general observation comes from Janie Bowthorpe, who wrote the *Stop the Thyroid Madness* book:

"Normally, a hypothyroid person is going to feel more refreshed when they wake up in the morning. So if someone doesn't feel that way, it's likely to be low adrenal function rather than low thyroid. A thyroid patient with no adrenal issues will generally wake up in the morning feeling okay and better refreshed. It's as the day progresses that it becomes clear how hypothyroid they are. Most of the time feeling un-refreshed first thing in the morning is far more likely to be a symptom of low cortisol, and feeing more tired in the afternoon is more likely to mean the thyroid patient has too little thyroid hormone...though having a cortisol problem can exacerbate the tiredness one feels as the morning progresses and when afternoon continues. The important thing is *first thing in the morning*. Even thyroid patients with the worst levels of hypothyroidism and without an adrenal issue, will feel more refreshed upon waking. So when someone says they are feeling un-refreshed upon waking, it's far more likely to be an adrenal problem than a hypothyroid problem based on patient experience over the years."

As covered in Chapter 11, it advisable to start the use of CT3M with relatively low levels of daytime thyroid medication. This is to avoid problems with symptoms caused by too high a daytime level. For instance, if before starting CT3M the thyroid patient is already on a high T3 or NDT dosage, but they report low body temperatures, feeling cold and tired, they almost certainly have more than enough thyroid hormone. These symptoms and signs could be due to either low cortisol, or else the overwhelming high level of T3 containing medication may be causing problems. Patient experience with CT3M has shown that sometimes symptoms and signs associated with hypothyroidism may be caused by excessive use of T3 or NDT in the daytime. These problems may worsen, or they may switch to more worrying symptoms associated with hyperthyroidism when a thyroid patient begins to use CT3M, as all this excess thyroid hormone may begin to be effective. As CT3M is started, body temperature, blood pressure, and heart rate may all rise alongside the appearance of other symptoms that suggest hyperthyroidism. **To avoid problems, it is often helpful when starting to use CT3M to be taking relatively low daytime doses of T3 containing thyroid medication.** Any medication or dosage changes should be discussed with the patient's own medical practitioner.

SYMPTOMS AND SIGNS TO MONITOR

The **main symptoms** that I tracked and recorded when recovering from thyroid disease included: mood; anxiety (including restlessness and irritability); mental ability and clarity; energy level; strength or weakness; digestive symptoms; skin condition; feeling warm or cold and muscle aches or pains.

The **main signs** that were tracked either by my doctor or by me were: resting heart rate; body temperature; resting blood pressure; weight gain or loss; blood sugar level; adrenal hormone test results; sex hormone test results; checking that the heart was working correctly (no abnormal rhythms or sounds); electrocardiogram (ECG); checking for evidence of bone loss; nutritional deficiencies and thyroid blood test results.

RECORDING SYMPTOMS AND SIGNS

It is extremely helpful for a thyroid patient to record symptoms and signs regularly, and in an organised way. Doing this makes it much easier to identify trends and to interpret what might be going on. It also provides excellent records to look back over. How this information is presented makes a great deal of difference to how easy it is to interpret.

Here is a good example of well-organised information that one thyroid patient recorded:

Date: 8th March 2011

Dosage: 25mcg@07:00; 12.5mcg@11:00; 12.5mcg@14:00; 12.5mcg@17:00.

Time since stopping using Thyroxine: 3 months (This is useful to record since it takes 8-12 weeks to fully clear excess T4, which in turn will lower reverse T3)

Get up time: 7:00 am

Signs:

TIME	TEMP	HR	BP
08:40:	36.7,	95,	107/64
10:00:	36.8,	97,	101/65
12:00:	36.8,	92,	105/63
13:40:	37.0,	97,	109/65
15:50:	37.0,	94,	109/66
18:00:	37.0,	92,	106/63

(If there had been any laboratory test results then these would be included, along with reference ranges - as laboratory test results are also *signs*).

Symptoms summary: Tired in the morning with headache. Didn't sleep well previous night. Felt warm from 12 noon & a bit on edge in the afternoon. Had energy in the afternoon, body feels 'lighter' & head feels clearer.

The above is clear, organised, and only has the essentials in it. This thyroid patient created a diary with time stamped (dated) entries with this type of information, which made it easy for her to track progress after any thyroid medication change (in this case it was T3 medication). It appeared that this individual had too high a heart rate, which she needed to discuss with her doctor and resolve through a thyroid medication adjustment, but it is easy to view the information.

Too much information, with many detailed descriptive comments, is almost as bad as too little; it can be very difficult to understand it. Summarising the symptoms and signs collected into a few lines makes it easy to create a diary that the thyroid patient and their doctor can easily assess. Pages of information with many detailed descriptive comments are much more difficult to use. When the information is summarised tidily, and in a short amount of space, then any obvious patterns or results may be found far more easily.

The type of thyroid medication being used, and the doses and timings, need to be recorded along with the signs (heart rate, body temperature and blood pressure, and any other laboratory test results). The time the thyroid patient gets up should also be recorded if they are using CT3M.

This type of diary or record can be a godsend when trying to understand what is happening. Often, only by looking at this information before and after changes to medication can some trend or situation be fully understood. It may seem a lot of work, but it is very useful. A diary like this can also be used to convince doctors that a safe and thorough approach is being taken with the use of thyroid medication.

SOME COMBINATIONS OF RESULTS TO LOOK FOR

Low body temperature, low blood pressure and low heart rate consistently over the day can often indicate low T3 or NDT thyroid hormones. These signs may be accompanied by an array of symptoms that suggest hypothyroidism. These may include: greater sense of pain (muscle and/or joint pain), tiredness, lack of motivation, brain fog or anxiety. The full list of symptoms associated with hypothyroidism is extensive. In this case it may be that the circadian dose is low, but it may also mean that the daytime thyroid medication is also too low.

High body temperature, elevated blood pressure and higher than normal heart rate may indicate an excess of thyroid hormones like T3 or NDT. These signs may be accompanied by shakiness, anxiety, agitation, weakness, a 'spacey' feeling, brain fog, muscle tightness (pain in neck, headache) and/or feeling physically overheated, or many other symptoms associated with excess thyroid hormone. Too much T3 or NDT thyroid hormone can raise the systolic blood pressure number (the first/top number), with diastolic blood pressure perhaps remaining the same or only slightly elevated. Too much thyroid hormone usually raises the heart rate and makes someone feel warmer (but this depends on whether there is enough cortisol and iron etc.). Anxiety and a feeling of tension/stress can also be caused by too much thyroid hormone, as can loose bowels.

SPECIFIC OBSERVATIONS ABOUT BODY TEMPERATURE

In this sub-section I refer to *basal temperature*. Basal temperature is the body temperature taken first thing when you awake, but before getting out of bed.[RWT3 2]

If the temperature is taken under the tongue, then a normal body temperature is 97.8 - 98.6 degrees Fahrenheit (36.5 - 37.0 degrees Centigrade). An under-the-armpit normal body temperature may be slightly lower at 97.8 - 98.2 degrees Fahrenheit (36.6 - 36.8 degrees Centigrade). Hypothyroid patients tend to have lower than normal body temperatures that often fall 1.5 - 3.0 degrees below normal on the Fahrenheit scale. **However, body temperature readings below 97.8 degrees Fahrenheit (36.6 degrees Centigrade) may suggest the presence of hypothyroidism, and this is the most important thing to remember.** Consequently, there should be great suspicion that a thyroid patient remains with some aspects of hypothyroidism if their body temperature is lower than 97.8 degrees Fahrenheit (36.6 degrees Centigrade).

Several body temperature readings should be taken over a period of days, ideally at the same time each day, in order to develop a clearer picture of how body temperature is varying.

If my body temperature readings were consistently below 98.0 degrees Fahrenheit (36.67 degrees Centigrade), then I suspected that my T3 dosage was too low. This is a little higher than the 97.8 degrees Fahrenheit (36.6 degrees Centigrade) which Dr. Barnes suggested, but this is what I personally found. Temperature readings consistently above 98.6 degrees Fahrenheit (37.0 degrees Centigrade) led me to suspect that my T3 had been over-replaced. Certainly, if my body temperature was lower than 97.8 degrees Fahrenheit (36.6 degrees Centigrade), then I strongly suspected that I was under-replaced. If my body temperature readings were in the 98.4 to 98.6 degrees Fahrenheit range (36.88 - 37.0 degrees Centigrade), then I usually felt well. This is where my temperature lies most of the time during the day now. This is quite a typical result for many correctly treated thyroid patients.

Frequently, body temperature may start the day lower and then improve as the day goes on. If this trend was present, then it can be helpful to take an average of the body temperature readings over the day. It is important not to conclude too much based on basal temperature though, as this is often much lower than body temperature during the daytime.

It is also important to note that, for women who are still having menstrual cycles, the basal temperature can vary across the month. However, for the purposes of CT3M assessment, temperature is just one measure, and this variation due to cycling is unlikely to be a major factor in applying CT3M correctly.

TAKING BODY TEMPERATURE READINGS WHEN USING CT3M

When trying to assess the success of the circadian dose, it is important to take a reading of body temperature within the first hour after rising. Readings of body temperature mid/late morning, mid/late afternoon and in the evening are also useful. More specifically, I'd suggest that at least three or four body temperature readings, combined with the recording of blood pressure, heart rate and symptoms over each day, are helpful when someone is trying to assess thyroid hormone effectiveness using symptoms and signs.

If several doses of T3 or NDT are being used over the day, it is often very effective to use the following approach:

- Take one body temperature reading during the first hour after getting up. This provides some assessment of the effectiveness of the circadian dose. This should be combined with a recording of blood pressure and heart rate. A brief note of relevant symptoms (or changes in symptoms) is also extremely helpful.

- Take a body temperature reading just before each daytime dose of thyroid medication (NDT or T3 dose). Heart rate, blood pressure and any significant symptoms should also be recorded. Recording symptoms and signs just before a T3 or NDT dose is due should provide useful information about whether the dose was due to be taken, or whether it might be too late.

- Take a body temperature reading two to three hours after each daytime dose of thyroid medication. Also, accompany this with the other suggested readings. This should provide helpful insight into the effectiveness of the daytime doses of thyroid medication and perhaps how well CT3M is beginning to work.

- If it is possible to do this, then repeating these measurements at the same times each day is useful so that a comparison can be made and any trends spotted. Several days of readings may be needed to draw any real conclusion.

- For thyroid patients using NDT, an average daytime temperature may be entirely adequate.

Temperatures can drop if you are very relaxed, sleepy (taking a nap), have had a recent shower or bath, or have been outside on a cold day. Eating and drinking also affect temperature readings, so waiting for at least fifteen minutes after food or drink is helpful.

SPECIFIC OBSERVATIONS ABOUT HEART RATE

Heart rate can often provide some clue about whether thyroid hormone dosage is too high or too low. Certainly, if a thyroid patient's heart rate is above 90 BPM (beats per minute) then there is a possibility that thyroid hormone dosage may be too high. If it is lower than 60 BPM, it is possible that thyroid hormone dosage is too low. These are just guidelines of course, and don't account for some individuals with unusual metabolisms or unique health issues not related to thyroid hormone. Typical healthy heart rate is often in the 65/70 - 80/85 BPM range.

If a thyroid patient finds that they have **a high heart rate, but low body temperature and low blood pressure, then this might be due to low thyroid hormone levels**, which can sometimes drive heart rate up. In this situation, when the next dose of NDT or T3 medication is taken, it may actually lower heart rate, and raise both blood pressure and body temperature. This response would tend to confirm the suspicion that the elevated heart rate is due to low thyroid hormone levels.

If a thyroid patient has **a low heart rate, but low body temperature and raised blood pressure, then this may also be an indicator of low thyroid hormone levels**. In this case, the next dose of T3 or NDT medication should normalise heart rate, lower blood pressure and raise body temperature.

High heart rate, with raised blood pressure, may be an indication of adrenaline production due to low cortisol that comes from partial adrenal insufficiency. In this situation, body temperature may be low, normal or even high because of the action of adrenaline. In this case, the heart rate is often well above 90, and blood pressure may be higher than normal for the individual.

Feeling as if the **heart is pounding with normal heart rate, body temperature and blood pressure might indicate the need for electrolytes** such as magnesium, potassium, or calcium or any combination of these. A fast pounding heart rate can be suggestive of low sodium.

A slow pounding heart with low (or raised) blood pressure and low body temperature could suggest low thyroid hormone levels.

A pounding heart can also be the effect of adrenaline due to low cortisol (this is often accompanied by raised blood pressure, but it depends on the severity of the low cortisol issue). The late Dr. John Lowe said if all vitals seem normal, a mild pounding sensation could be a sign of adequate thyroid hormone levels as thyroid patients are not used to the normal healthy heart beat.

REMINDER OF SYMPTOMS ASSOCIATED WITH ADRENAL ISSUES

These lists come directly out of the *Recovering with T3* book. I felt it would be helpful to include these in this chapter.

There are some clues when cortisol insufficiency is present:
- Low blood sugar, which may cause dizziness, feeling unwell or more frequent hunger.
- Severe fatigue/tiredness.
- Aches and pains.
- Dizziness (even when sitting down).
- Clumsiness.

- Poor response to thyroid hormone replacement therapy.
- Anxiousness or inability to cope with stress.
- Irritability or anger or panic feelings.
- Feeling cold/low body temperature.
- Fluctuating body temperature. Some doctors in the USA ask their thyroid patients to take body temperature readings three hours after waking, three hours later and a further three hours after that. These are averaged for the day to form the daily average body temperature (DAT). If a thyroid patient's DAT varies more than 0.2 degrees Fahrenheit, then this may suggest cortisol insufficiency when combined with other evidence.
- Possibly having dark rings under the eyes.
- Pale and 'washed out' skin colour, or even a slight darkening of the skin.
- Skin appears thinner.
- Digestive upsets, which may including diarrhoea.
- Worsening allergies.
- Symptoms similar to a flu virus.
- Nausea.
- Trembling, shakiness or a jittery/hyper feeling.
- Rapid heartbeat or pounding.
- Difficulty sleeping.
- Low blood pressure as a result of the impact on the action of thyroid hormones.
- Low back pain - where the adrenal glands are located.
- Worsening symptoms in the presence of stress of any kind, including minor infections.

There are some clues when aldosterone insufficiency is present:
- Low blood pressure, which is even lower if the blood pressure is taken immediately after the patient stands up (postural hypotension).
- Craving for salty foods.
- Thirst.
- Dizziness when standing up, which may include fainting.
- More frequent need to urinate, or frequent urination during the night.
- Excessive sweating.
- A slightly higher body temperature than usual.
- High heart rate.

Low levels of thyroid hormone can also cause several of the above symptoms. This can obviously make recognising adrenal insufficiency a bit of a challenge. It is extremely helpful to have a twenty-four hour adrenal saliva test to confirm actual cortisol status.

There are some clues when high cortisol is present:
- High blood pressure.
- Bruising easily.
- Fluid retention.
- Obesity and/or moon-shaped face, increased belly fat, fat on the back of the neck.
- Fatigue.
- Weak muscles and muscle loss.

There are some clues when high aldosterone is present:
- High blood pressure.
- Low potassium - which can cause weakness or muscle spasms.
- Numbness, or tingling in the extremities.
- Frequent urination.

FINAL COMMENTS

In addition to all the above, it is very important to look at trends and changes that have occurred due to dosage changes of thyroid medication. Often, the **most important information** may be found by assessing changes to the circadian dose or daytime dose of thyroid medication, that has caused changes in the symptoms and signs. Very often just looking at heart rate, body temperature and blood pressure alone at any given time will not be enough to assess what should be done to improve adrenal function and symptoms and signs. However, by looking at **responses to the changes in thyroid medication** a far clearer picture of what is occurring may be revealed.

Finally, repeating laboratory testing of cortisol, iron or other nutrients, hormones, or values that are important for the individual patient, may also be required. This may provide insight into what is happening with thyroid hormone action and the partial adrenal insufficiency that CT3M is seeking to address.

As with most other comments within this book, the thyroid patient should discuss any medication or dosage changes with their own doctor.

Chapter 17

Restarting CT3M

This is a brief, but very important chapter. In trying to establish the optimal thyroid medication solution, various changes will be made to dosages and/or to the timing of taking these. Often, such changes will result in changes to symptoms and signs that are easy to interpret, and with common sense the thyroid patient and doctor will know what to do next. However, in other situations, the results of the changes may be poor or confusing, or both, resulting in immense head scratching. Neither patient nor doctor may know what is going on, or why the changes that they thought were going to be effective have actually resulted in a poor response. This situation can arise from making changes too quickly, and not waiting for enough time to really observe the effect of the last change!

Patience is needed when thyroid doses are adjusted. The adrenal glands take time to fully adjust, and raising doses of thyroid medication, or adjusting the time they are taken too frequently, will just cause confusion.

There are two responses that can be taken at this point, and both are immensely useful:

- Revert back to the last known best-case dosage of thyroid hormone and CT3M dosage/timing.
- Restart CT3M.

REVERTING TO THE LAST GOOD DOSAGE OF THYROID HORMONE AND CT3M DOSAGE/TIMING

This is something I myself had to do quite often. Even with very careful recording and assessment of symptoms and signs, sometimes the choice over what thyroid medication change to make can be difficult. Inevitably, from time-to-time a poor choice will be made, and the thyroid patient will feel slightly worse or considerably worse after the change. This may apply to either a timing or dosage change to the circadian dose, or to one of the daytime doses. If several dosage changes have been made over several weeks, there may have been more than one alteration in dosage or timing that have combined to produce a less than effective result.

In these situations, the best solution is often to review the recorded notes on symptoms and signs over time, and revert back to a dosage and timing of the circadian and daytime doses that have worked more effectively. This may mean reverting back to a dosage used several weeks, or even months earlier.

To some thyroid patients, reverting back to a previous dosage may feel like a failure, but it isn't. Getting to a known, stable dosage provides a more stable platform from which to assess any further CT3M or daytime thyroid medication changes. Any future changes may also be made with the knowledge of which changes did not work, and this can help to provide a better understanding of what is actually going on.

This strategy of reverting back to a previous stable dosage/timing of CT3M and daytime thyroid medication should be employed a lot more often, I suspect. It can really help, and..... it isn't a failure!

RESTARTING CT3M

In some situations, it makes sense to completely restart CT3M with a small dose of T3 or NDT taken at 1.5 hours before getting up, i.e. a complete restart of CT3M. This is a good strategy if there have been substantial changes. These changes might include:

- A change of thyroid medication type, e.g. switching the circadian dose to T3 from NDT, or changing the daytime doses from NDT to T3 (or from T4 to NDT).
- A large improvement in a nutrient that was deficient, e.g. iron levels that are now optimal.
- After other medications have been added or removed, e.g. if someone has been using LDN (low dose naltrexone) for some time.
- After the weaning of adrenal glandulars or adrenal steroids. It is very important to restart CT3M after this, as the situation with respect to adrenal hormones may have changed significantly.
- If the thyroid patient and their doctor have become very confused over what is happening, and do not know what previous dosage to revert back to.
- Over time, the adrenal glands may improve substantially and the thyroid patient may feel significantly healthier. The patient and their doctor may decide to keep a note of the current thyroid medication dosage and CT3M dosage/timing. They may then try applying CT3M from the start to see how much of an improvement in adrenal performance has occurred. Sometimes, only by a complete re-start might this be discovered.

Restarting CT3M is a very useful strategy, and one that I have occasionally used in the past. It is an essential approach after significant medication changes, e.g. after weaning adrenal steroids.

As with all medication changes mentioned within this book, the thyroid patient should be discussing these with their own personal physician.

Chapter 18

Adrenal Steroids and CT3M

It is critical to be aware that some people cannot manage without taking their adrenal hormones. For people with Addison's disease, or other conditions that dramatically affect the capability of the adrenal glands, there is simply no option but to take adrenal hormones. Hypopituitarism is another condition for which adrenal hormones have to be taken. Some inflammatory conditions also require the permanent use of adrenal steroids.

Many patients I have spoken to who have applied CT3M, have improved their adrenal function and have addressed their issues with partial adrenal insufficiency. In many cases, the amazingly simple CT3M concept has allowed patients to **slowly** wean themselves from the use of adrenal glandulars or adrenal steroids under the guidance of their doctor.

There are various articles available on the Internet that discuss the merits of providing low levels of adrenal hormones for a short while during thyroid hormone treatment. These articles invariably state that this should only be done for a short period of time. Then, once the thyroid hormone treatment is working, the adrenal hormones should gradually be reduced, then stopped. However, many patients still appear to be on adrenal hormones after several years have passed by. It is also useful to think about why most of these thyroid patients have so easily passed a Synacthen Test (or ACTH Stimulation Test) in the past.

Numerous thyroid patients all over the world have now used CT3M. An increasing amount of evidence from patient experience has now become available. Large numbers of these thyroid patients have responded well to CT3M. In some cases, other health issues have also been corrected before CT3M could work effectively.

The conclusion I have reached from the above, is that a majority of thyroid patients with partial adrenal insufficiency have this problem as a secondary consequence to hypothyroidism. The partial adrenal insufficiency may have been made worse by issues such as immune system stresses, gut flora imbalances, nutrient problems, toxicity or stress. However, in the majority of people, partial adrenal insufficiency is occurring due to low free T3 levels that have been present for too long as a result of inadequate treatment for hypothyroidism. The inadequate treatment may have arisen from the use of levothyroxine (T4), which is frequently a poor treatment choice, or from not allowing the patient's FT3 levels to rise enough (perhaps by placing far too much emphasis on TSH laboratory testing). In some cases, thyroid patients may not have been diagnosed with hypothyroidism, yet they may have had this problem for many years. Long-term poor treatment for hypothyroidism using levothyroxine (T4), is believed by many of us to lead to lower than healthy FT3 levels and other chronic health conditions. It is this combination of chronic health issues and low FT3 that I am convinced leads to the partial adrenal insufficiency.

The good results that have been seen with CT3M have surprised me. I never expected CT3M to be as widely applicable as it has turned out to be. This has convinced me that most people suffering with partial adrenal insufficiency (adrenal fatigue) do not have damaged or even 'tired' adrenal glands. All that is needed is for more T3 to be available to support the adrenal glands when they need to produce a high volume of cortisol, combined with a focus on any other health issues that may be causing problems, i.e. a more holistic approach to the health of the thyroid patient.

I do not believe that most thyroid patients who are using adrenal glandulars or adrenal steroids have 'tired adrenals' or 'damaged adrenal glands' at all. I also don't believe that using adrenal glandulars or adrenal steroids 'rests tired adrenals'. Perhaps this is why so many people that start using adrenal steroids simply cannot get off them again. These drugs should rarely be given, apart from Addison's disease (proven via a Synacthen test, adrenal autoantibody testing or an adrenal gland scan) and hypopituitarism (proven via an insulin tolerance test).

Once adrenal glandulars or adrenal steroids have been used for a long time, it is possible to become reliant on them. The effect is to reduce the demand from the pituitary/hypothalamus to the adrenal glands, and for the adrenal glands to become more sluggish and less able to cope. These adrenal glandulars and adrenal steroids should be a last resort, not a first line option.

I believe CT3M should be the first choice of treatment for partial adrenal insufficiency if there is no underlying adrenal or HPA axis issue that would necessitate the use of adrenal steroids (no Addison's Disease or hypopituitarism). When combined with an overall approach to the health of the thyroid patient, and the resolution of other chronic health issues, CT3M provides a good option in the toolkit for the treatment of partial adrenal insufficiency.

WHAT IF A THYROID PATIENT IS ALREADY ON ADRENAL GLANDULARS OR ADRENAL STEROIDS LIKE HYDROCORTISONE OR FLORINEF?

Some people believe that CT3M is not applicable for a thyroid patient who is already taking adrenal glandulars or adrenal steroids. This is not true. There are three options that are possible:

1. **Wean the adrenal steroids or adrenal glandulars before starting CT3M.** This option is only applicable if the thyroid patient is on a very low dose of adrenal steroids or glandulars, or feels that these have not helped them at all. The

advantages are that this makes applying CT3M simpler and easier to monitor, as any adrenal support has already been removed. The thyroid patient should discuss this option with their own doctor and decide if it is the best option for them.

2.   **Wean the adrenal steroids or adrenal glandulars as CT3M is applied.** This is applicable if the thyroid patient is taking a low to moderate dose of adrenal steroids/glandulars, and the patient's doctor feels it is not safe to wean the steroids without also adding in CT3M. This is by far the most frequent option selected when CT3M is needed for a thyroid patient who is using adrenal glandulars or adrenal steroids.

3.   **Apply CT3M as an additional support alongside adrenal glandulars or adrenal steroids.** This option is only really sensible for those patients who have already received a diagnosis of Addison's disease or hypopituitarism. These patients have to use adrenal steroids or glandulars. Some of these patients have had success when they have also added CT3M into their regime. This is not a result I would ever have predicted, but for some at least it appears to help. I suspect these patients who have benefited must have had some remaining adrenal function.

I will now get off my soapbox and leave this chapter as the preamble for the following one, which discusses how a thyroid patient might wean themselves off adrenal steroids/glandulars when starting CT3M.

Chapter 19

Observations on Weaning Adrenal Steroids

The information within this chapter has been obtained directly from the experience of thyroid patients who have weaned adrenal glandulars and adrenal steroids whilst applying CT3M.

This chapter is only relevant to those thyroid patients who have no fundamental adrenal damage, no hypopituitarism and are not taking steroids for the treatment of some other health condition. It is also extremely important that any weaning of adrenal steroids is carried out under the supervision of a qualified medical practitioner.

When using CT3M, adrenal hormones should be weaned in order to allow the adrenals to receive an adequate request from the body to make adrenal hormones. For cortisol, this request arrives in the form of ACTH from the pituitary. Whilst adrenal hormones are being taken, then CT3M may not work fully. Consequently, the adrenals themselves may not have the right environment to improve their production of hormones. I sometimes say that the adrenal steroids are the *lullaby that sings the adrenals to sleep*. This is clearly not true for all thyroid patients, as some definitely do require adrenal steroids and obtain a benefit from them.

CT3M can be described to people as a *very clean process*; it only requires the thyroid medication (T3 or NDT) that someone may already be using to implement it. It requires no other drugs, just common sense and patience.

In many cases, if CT3M were offered as the first choice treatment for partial adrenal insufficiency for thyroid patients, then it is likely that they would avoid ever having to consider the use of adrenal glandulars or adrenal steroids like hydrocortisone or Florinef.

At the same time as using CT3M (as described in Chapter 11), the following process for weaning adrenal glandulars/steroids may also be used:

APPROACH TO WEANING ADRENAL STEROIDS STEP BY STEP

If a thyroid patient is already on adrenal hormones when CT3M is applied, then the approach described here for weaning these has been seen to be successful. It is based on the experience of many thyroid patients, but it should also be carried out with the support of the patient's own personal physician:

1. No adrenal steroids should be taken within the main cortisol production window (i.e. the last four hours of sleep). Consequently, the first dose of any adrenal medication should be taken no earlier than when the thyroid patient gets up in the morning (ideally at least an hour or two later than this). This is to give the adrenal glands a chance to respond to the circadian dose.

2. **Florinef weaning.** All Florinef (which is the synthetic equivalent of aldosterone), and all slow potassium, should be weaned first. This is before any attempt is made to reduce cortisol-containing medication (hydrocortisone or prednisolone). Florinef affects blood pressure too much to be left in place as the circadian dose is titrated. High blood pressure may result if CT3M is applied without weaning Florinef at the same time.

3. Thyroid patients have found that Florinef should be weaned in stages, with a small fraction of the Florinef being removed at a time as CT3M is applied. Florinef depresses potassium, and if someone is taking slow release potassium then this needs to be reduced at the same time that the Florinef is weaned.

4. Good results have been seen when Florinef is weaned by quarter tablet reductions, sometimes reducing by a half a tablet every week (1 tablet is 0.1mg of Florinef). Slow potassium should be weaned in proportion. For example, for someone on half a tablet of Florinef and 16 MEQ of slow-K, they may wean to a quarter of a tablet of Florinef and at the same time reduce their slow-K to 8 MEQ (MEQ stands for milliequivalent). If the Florinef remains too high when CT3M is applied, then it will raise blood pressure very quickly after taking it. By tracking symptoms and signs it should be possible to manage the weaning process as CT3M is applied.

5. CT3M may be started, and the circadian dose adjusted (i.e. dose time and size), as the Florinef and any potassium medication is fully weaned. This may need the support of the patient's doctor. At the very least, the patient's own medical practitioner should be aware of this process and be available to support the patient. Once a circadian dose has been found that seems to help, then many patients have found it useful not to change that dose during the weaning of adrenal steroids, as too many changes can be confusing and unnecessary.

6. If high blood pressure is present during the weaning of Florinef, then the weaning of hydrocortisone (HC) or any cortisol containing medication should be started at the same time (see points 7 - 10). In this case, the first HC dose should be the focus of weaning (points 8 - 9).

7. **Hydrocortisone weaning**. Once all Florinef and any slow potassium are weaned, the next task is to remove cortisol-containing medication, such as hydrocortisone (HC). HC depresses potassium, and this is another reason to wean all slow potassium before any HC is reduced.

8. HC is normally taken in divided doses during the day. The following three approaches have been seen to work well:

a) The first HC dose of the day (which must not be taken during the last four hours of sleep), is delayed or pushed forward in time. Ideally, the delay should be for as long as feels comfortably possible. If the delay is long enough for the second HC dose to be due, this first HC dose may be dropped completely. This may occur immediately if the response to CT3M is good. If the first HC dose is still needed before the second HC dose is due, then the first HC dose is trimmed by at least 2.5 mg.

b) An alternative is to begin by weaning the first HC dose of the day and, at the same time, move this trimmed HC dose to later in the day. Every day or two, the first dose of HC may be moved an hour or so later. It should be trimmed by at least 2.5 mg each day if possible. Eventually, the first HC dose will be close to the second HC dose, and may be dropped totally.

c) The third approach to weaning HC is to delay the first HC dose by as much as is comfortable, and to delay all the other HC doses by the same amount of time. In this approach, the last HC dose of the day will end up being later in the day, and will be reduced by at least 2.5 mg every time the movement of the doses occur. This approach may be relevant if the thyroid patient appears to need both the first and second HC doses to remain at the same levels for a little longer whilst the circadian dose is adjusted.

9. By moving the first dose of HC to a later time, this creates more time during which the adrenal glands are required to support the patient's body on their own (with no suppressive effect from HC via any lowering of ACTH from the pituitary). This movement later in time of the first dose of HC, and the frequent cutting of it by 2.5 mg, really allows the adrenal glands freedom to work correctly. As the HC weaning progresses, the circadian dose is adjusted further if needed.

10. Once the first HC dose has been moved and effectively dropped, the remaining doses of HC may be weaned by 2.5 mg (or more) each day. Eventually, when there is only 10mg of HC adrenal medication being used, often it may be stopped completely.

11. **General Observations on weaning of adrenal steroids.** It is worth pointing out that during the weaning of steroids, that sometimes when a dose of HC or Florinef (or adrenal glandulars if these are being used) is taken, this may produce very marked adverse symptoms. An example of this might be extreme nausea following a dose of HC or Florinef. When noticeably adverse symptoms occur, this may also provide excellent information suggesting that the adrenal steroid dose is ready to be weaned further.

12. CT3M should be enabling the adrenal glands to work well enough on their own at this point, but further titration of the circadian dose may be required. In some cases, when no steroid medication is being used, the response to the circadian dose may be too potent because of the suppressive effect that the steroids were previously having on the adrenal glands.

13. Following the process of slow weaning and stopping all adrenal steroids, if symptoms and signs are not normal and do not suggest good adrenal function, CT3M should be re-started (as covered in Chapter 17). This means restarting with a low dose of T3 (possibly 10-micrograms) or NDT (1 grain), 1.5 hours before the time that the thyroid patient gets up. Adjusting the circadian dose fully with no steroids present often resolves any remaining issues. This may need to be repeated over time as the adrenal glands improve their production. It is important to allow several days in between each change to the circadian dose to ensure the effects can be assessed.

14. This weaning process does not need to take months and months - four weeks is often sufficient. However, the adrenal glands may not fully recover immediately, and a circadian dose may need to be found that supports the adrenals without over-stressing them. Over time the adrenal glands should improve their production of cortisol and other hormones. It is advisable to re-take a twenty-four hour adrenal saliva test from time to time. In some cases, the circadian dose of T3 may need to be fine-tuned further. If there is any doubt over what is going on, a **re-start of CT3M** may be required, i.e. by using a low dose of T3-containing medication taken at 1.5 hours before getting up.

The process outlined above is based on the experience of many thyroid patients who have applied CT3M and, at the same time, successfully weaned themselves from adrenal steroids. Patients using adrenal glandulars may be treated in accordance with the above HC weaning guidelines, with the first adrenal glandular dose being weaned first (i.e. steps 8 – 10 above).

The above process appears to work well, but inevitably it may not be a smooth process due to the powerful nature of adrenal steroids. The process will be far easier if there is good support from a doctor, or from other thyroid patients who have been through this themselves.

It is also important to be aware that even after all steroids have been weaned, the adrenal glands may take a considerable amount of time (weeks or months) to respond well. During this time, more adjustment may be required to the circadian dose.

Applying CT3M and weaning from adrenal steroids may need to be combined with other diagnostic and treatment approaches if the thyroid patient has any underlying health issues.

Chapter 20

Bedtime Doses of T3/NDT and Use of LDN

Some thyroid patients find that even after applying CT3M and optimising the circadian dose, that their cortisol levels are still not optimal. The situations and conditions that can undermine CT3M (Chapter 8) should be reviewed before considering bedtime doses of T3 or NDT, or LDN use. However, bedtime doses of thyroid medication and LDN use can both be profoundly helpful for some thyroid patients. Let me discuss both of these options a little further.

BEDTIME DOSE OF T3 OR NDT

For those thyroid patients who find that they need a little more help with adrenal function after several months of applying CT3M, then the use of a small bedtime dose of T3 (perhaps 2.5, 5 or even 10 micrograms of T3), or the equivalent of NDT, may be tried. This seems to prepare the adrenals for the use of CT3M for some patients. Whether this bedtime dose is helping the HPA axis, or is having a direct effect on the adrenal glands, is not clear. However, what is clear is that for some thyroid patients it is another piece of the puzzle that may need to be put in place.

The caution here is that for some thyroid patients, a bedtime dose creates tissue over-stimulation (either during the night, or during the next day) when combined with CT3M. Bedtime use of T3 or NDT can actually destabilise CT3M, and make further progress much more difficult. This is why it is suggested that everything that can possibly be done to fine-tune both CT3M and daytime thyroid medication should be tried before considering bedtime dosing with T3 or NDT.

The use of a bedtime dose of T3-containing medication may require further fine-tuning of CT3M and daytime thyroid medication. It may take several weeks to re-adjust any thyroid medication once the bedtime dose is introduced. However, for some thyroid patients it works well and can provide the final improvement step that they need. I prefer to see thyroid patients and their doctors consider this option after all other reasonable steps have been taken.

LOW DOSE NALTREXONE (LDN)

I know of a number of thyroid patients who have experienced significant improvements in their cortisol levels with the use of CT3M, but have still not quite managed to improve the function of their adrenals to the level that made them feel really healthy. Some of these patients have then gone on to work with their own doctors to trial LDN.

Naltrexone is an opioid antagonist that has been used and approved to treat opioid addiction and alcohol addiction - at high doses (50 mg a day). When naltrexone is taken in low doses (0.5 - 4.5 mg a day), it is known as low dose naltrexone (or LDN). LDN has been shown by researchers to work in a different way to naltrexone. LDN is believed to stimulate the production of more endorphins, which modulate the immune system and re-balance any excessive immune system responses through its effect on opioid receptors. LDN is only used in low doses. The starting dose of LDN is frequently 0.5, 1 or 1.5 milligrams. This daily dose, often taken at bedtime is sometimes raised slowly over months. It is raised until a level is found that improves symptoms, but no higher than a maximum of 4.5 milligrams. Some thyroid patients are very sensitive to LDN, and I know of several who get a good response from only 0.5 milligrams of LDN, being unable to tolerate a higher dose than this. This latter point is one reason why some doctors use a starting dose of LDN of 0.5 milligrams. I said that LDN is often taken at bedtime but it is worth noting that I also know of patients that take the LDN dose in the morning, or at a fixed time during the day (often due to sleeping issues that can follow a bedtime dose of LDN). I am also aware of quite a few patients who find it helpful to take the LDN at the same time as their circadian dose.

LDN is primarily used to treat some autoimmune diseases, including rheumatoid arthritis, multiple sclerosis and Crohn's disease. However, LDN also appears to have positive effects on adrenal performance, perhaps by its effect on the HPA axis, or possibly due to its effect on reducing pro-inflammatory cytokines. It would be helpful for more research work to be carried out to fully understand the mechanism involved in LDN's effect on cortisol levels.

From patient experience, it is extremely clear to me that LDN can often be the final step that a thyroid patient may need to take to improve their adrenal performance.

LDN is a prescription drug that may need the support of a helpful and open-minded doctor in order to obtain it under prescription. However, the side effects are rare, and provided that very low doses are used and carefully monitored, LDN can be an excellent option for a thyroid patient who needs a little more help in achieving adequate adrenal performance.

LDN use is something I would not suggest considering for a thyroid patient who does not have a serious autoimmune issue, at least until all other options for improving adrenal performance have been explored. It should be one of the last things to consider, simply because it may not be needed, and taking another prescription drug for life is not a good solution if it can be avoided.

Chapter 21

The Time Factor

Thyroid patients do not become ill overnight. Hypothyroidism creeps up on people until the symptoms are eventually bad enough to make them visit a doctor. Adrenal problems in particular can take months or years to develop due to prolonged or inadequately treated hypothyroidism, stress, gut issues, or other diseases or conditions. The use of the rarely effective T4 treatment for hypothyroidism is in many cases the major culprit in prolonging the symptoms of hypothyroidism and, after more time, partial adrenal insufficiency can develop.

During the process of becoming ill with hypothyroidism and adrenal issues, other chronic health issues can develop. In some cases, these other health issues may have been instrumental in causing the thyroid problems in the first place.

It takes a long time to become ill with thyroid and adrenal issues, and it may take some time to get well again.

My own health improved significantly when I developed and then began to use CT3M. With CT3M I became well enough to function relatively normally once again. However, further improvements took place over a period of years after I began to use CT3M. These occurred without me needing to make any specific CT3M dosage or timing changes. I believe that the continued improvements in my health were due to gradual increased performance in adrenal function that came about because my adrenal glands were being properly supported with T3 thyroid hormone. CT3M and patience was what I needed, and my own body did the rest of the work.

It is a common issue for thyroid patients to notice a positive response to CT3M, but not achieve an immediate and full recovery of their health. In these situations the answer is often *time*. Adrenal issues develop over time and it isn't reasonable to expect instant recovery. Once CT3M is in place, it may well take a long time for slow recovery to fully occur. CT3M may not have been applied correctly of course, and advice and input should be solicited on this. Having the support of a knowledgeable and empathetic doctor can be a huge help to thyroid patients during this process, as can revisiting the situations and conditions that can disrupt CT3M that are outlined in Chapter 8.

THINGS MAY CHANGE OVER TIME

Once the thyroid patient is on an effective circadian dose and appropriate daytime dose(s) of thyroid medication, then these may not remain precisely the same over time. Over months or years, as further improvement in adrenal performance occurs, further refinement of the size or timing of the circadian dose or daytime doses may be needed.

I know of some people who have reduced total T3 medication from quite high doses to just 10-15 mcg per day. Some only need a 5-10 mcg circadian dose. Others remain on their dosage at a stable level. Some find that they can move the circadian dose later in time i.e. closer to getting-up time. In a few cases, thyroid patients may be able to stop using CT3M altogether, as their adrenal glands may perform well enough without it. However, it may take many weeks after a reduction in a circadian dose, or stopping it completely, before it is clear if the adrenal glands are capable of producing enough cortisol without CT3M.

It is well over fifteen years since I began to use CT3M, and I still require it. I take 25 micrograms of T3 at 4:00 am now, which appears to be reasonably stable for me. I take two further doses of T3 during the daytime (20 micrograms at 11:30 am and 10 micrograms at 4:30 pm), which is also stable in my case. However, I know of others who have dramatically reduced their circadian dose and a few that no longer need it.

There is no *one size fits all* answer on whether thyroid patients will be able to stop using CT3M over time. Some will be able to stop using CT3M, and some will not feel as healthy without it. It is not possible to tell in advance whether someone will or won't be able to stop CT3M over time - only time will show this.

For those thyroid patients, like me, who continue to require CT3M, then I do not see this as a hardship at all. Provided there is adequate preparation, it is easy to take a circadian dose in total darkness (with speed and simplicity), and then fall back to a deep and high quality sleep.

SECTION 3

WRAPPING UP

,

Chapter 22

Thyroid Patient Experience with CT3M

These stories have very kindly been given to me by thyroid patients. They talk about how CT3M has changed their health and lives.

Each story is followed by a few observations of my own.

SUE'S STORY

Briefly, I suffered from hypo symptoms for about 20 years. Blood tests were always 'in range', and I've been diagnosed by various GPs in the past as depressed, fat, lazy, obsessive and having 'early stage CFS'. I became fatigued in 2008 and unable to function due to pain and exhaustion. I researched my symptoms, and everything pointed to hypothyroidism. After joining an online hypo forum, and seeking the advice of a private thyroid specialist, I firstly tried NDT. When this made me toxic, I went onto T3 only (62.5 mcg split into 3 doses taken at 8 am, 2 pm, 6 pm). This, at the time, was supplemented with Prednisolone (5 mcg), as my adrenal tests showed very low cortisol levels.

I improved significantly on this protocol, but I wasn't brimming with energy. I had good days and bad days. It was whilst I was on holiday that I remembered reading your views on taking T3 early in the morning, and because I was waking early with the Spanish sun shining through my window, I gave it a go. I had an instant improvement, didn't need to sleep in the afternoon, and even went walking in the hills on a couple of occasions. I stopped the Prednisolone pretty much within a week (not advisable, I know), but my body simply said that I didn't need it. My doses were 25 mcg T3 at 4.45 am, 25 mcg at 1 pm and 12.5mcg at 6 pm. I was walking 3 miles every day for the next few weeks, feeling absolutely marvelous, and for the first time in decades could remember what having boundless energy felt like.

Disappointingly, I started to struggle after a few months, and then spent the next 9 months titrating my doses until I arrived at what now feels like my ideal protocol. My doses have reduced dramatically, and I now take 6.25 mcg (a quarter tablet of T3) at 4.30 am and 6.25 mcg at 10.30 am.

Very occasionally I take another 6.25 mcg at 4:30 pm, but only if I feel a bit dodgy.

In June I swam a lake for charity. I've also written two novels in the last 12 months. Today I moved the furniture out of my bedroom, painted the walls and put the whole lot back in again. I have my eye on a triathlon next year. I cannot begin to express my excitement and relief at getting the best days of my life back thanks to you and your CT3M protocol. Had you not suffered, researched, battled and shared your life story, I would still be living a 'half-life' believing I was a fat, lazy, depressed failure. I'm so grateful to you Paul.

Two months ago, I woke up one day and knew I could at last lose weight. My body often tells my mind when it's ready for change! I'm on my own version of the paleo diet, having pretty much cut out non-nutritious carbs, including wheat (dire cold-turkey withdrawal, but worth the agony!). I never knew I had a gluten problem until I gave it up. I'm 28 pounds lighter, not hungry, not craving anything. In fact, I'm a fat burning machine! I'm lifting weights and starting to look great (still a long way to go). But everything those GPs said to me about being lazy and greedy, about having no willpower and driving myself into a diabetic, coronary early grave, was hogwash. I sort of always knew it, but didn't have a solution. Now I have - it's CT3M.

I have never had a hypo diagnosis through a blood test. Yet 12.5 mcg of T3 has transformed my health. It took 4 years to find the answer, but every step was vitally important. The missing key, which took me from nearly well to really well, was CT3M.

Thanks Paul. As Ghandi said, "First they ignore you, then they laugh at you, then they listen." I look forward to the day that doctors listen to you, so that everyone can feel the way I do now.

Keep up the fight!

I asked Sue how she had arrived at the low T3 doses, and this is the interesting reply she gave me:

The issue I had with my T3 dosing was that my blood pressure was always high (ish), even though I had hypo symptoms. I experimented for a while, but when I stepped back and thought about it, I decided that the blood pressure was the significant factor. I also remembered a doctor saying to me that if you take too much T3 your body sometimes "shuts down" to protect itself. Logic then told me that I was taking too much (blood pressure was the clue) and my body was shutting down (hypo symptoms). On this basis I gradually reduced my dose over a period of a few months. The hypo symptoms lessened and I felt better.

I continued with this until I was taking nothing. After a few days of zero T3, I felt like I was "walking off a cliff". Not a good feeling. I therefore took a small dose of 6.25 mcg at 4.45 am (always my optimum timing), and felt better immediately. I experimented with a second dose, eventually settling at 6.25 mcg at 10.30 am (almost 6 hours after the first dose). I sometimes get palpitations around 7-8 pm, and, if I do, I make a point of adding a third dose of 6.25 mcg at 4 pm the next day. Usually I can identify what has caused me to need the third dose - things like late nights, heavy exercise, swimming freezing lakes etc!

The other thing that catapulted me into amazing levels of energy was cutting carbohydrate out of my diet. I've been on the paleo diet for months, but I always struggled to stick to it consistently. The day I woke up and thought, "I'm fixed", I knew I could now lose the weight. Having said that, the withdrawal from sugar, grains and gluten was horrific for 5 days, and I wouldn't wish it on anyone. The fact that I was able to stick with it showed a massive difference in my metabolism. The thyroid hormone was exactly where it should be, the energy train was working and the gluten problem I didn't know I had was being rectified. After 5 days my headache went, and I coughed my lungs up all day (odd, but must've been something to do with the gluten?). Since then I've felt amazing, and I am losing weight easily. I have a lot to lose, but everything works the way it should now.

I guess the other conclusion I've drawn is that the problem for me was probably exhausted adrenals more than any massive thyroid problem. Once my adrenals got a bit of T3 at the time they needed it, my health came flooding back. Which is why I'm getting away with such a small dose of T3. There may come a time when I don't need it at all? Also, I suspect my need for T3 links to my peak requirement for cortisol, i.e. early morning and before 1 pm. Again, this may mean I won't need T3 forever. I never stood a chance of getting this diagnosed by a GP or endocrinologist. I believe that there are thousands of fat and knackered middle-aged women enduring the 'half-life' that I had. I'm literally buzzing with energy these days. I couldn't have wished for or imagined it was possible to feel this way!

I changed my T3 dose a little in November 2012 - now I'm taking 12.5 mcg at 4.45 am (circadian dose as part of CT3M), plus 6.25 mcg at 10.45 am. I get up at 6.45 am, which means my circadian dose is taken 2 hours before I get up.

Very occasionally I'll add an afternoon dose (6.25 mcg at 4.45 pm), but only if I'm clearly hypo. I was experiencing a little bit of headachy tiredness upon waking, so I upped the early morning T3 from 6.25 mcg to 12.5 mcg and it did the trick.

Also, I've lost 3 stones in weight since September 2012, and just recently met a wonderful man to whom I'm now engaged (hence the hectic lifestyle just now).

One of the main things I've noticed, having now got my condition under control, is that as the thyroid symptoms ease, other symptoms come to the fore. I'm currently using natural progesterone cream to tackle lingering PMS symptoms, with some encouraging results. I'm obsessive about the food I eat and things I choose to put on my skin - all as natural as possible.

I remain deeply suspicious and distrustful of the medical profession, and have full and total control over my own health. I dread to think where I would be now if I hadn't sought an alternative to the NHS's dismissal of my health!

Paul's Observations: I think Sue's story is fascinating for four reasons:
1. A few thyroid patients will only need a relatively small amount of T3 or NDT

medication to correct their health issues. It does not always need 40 micrograms of T3 (or more), or the equivalent in NDT, in order to recover.

2. Some thyroid patients may have more issues with partial adrenal insufficiency than they do with thyroid hormone imbalances. In these cases, emphasis on CT3M with minimal daytime dosing (or none) of thyroid medication can be what is needed.

3. Very often thyroid patients do not make a full recovery without addressing many other health issues, such as sex hormones. Gut health and diet is usually high up the list. Sue is a classic example of this, and without her attention, focus and sheer determination to improve her health in many areas, she would not have achieved the absolutely fantastic results that she has.

4. Finally, many people and their doctors believe that they will have to accept a poor quality of health. It is not unusual to hear of patients who have been told that at their age, they just need to accept that they will have problems, or be exhausted, or be overweight. This is nonsense, and is often a very poor excuse on the part of the doctor who has said it. I was told that I would have to put up with my own symptoms and just live with the situation. Sue's case is yet another example of what can be achieved when the entire health of the person is looked at and improved. CT3M was obviously a key part of that, but the focus on overall total health was critical.

MARY'S STORY

This is my story of how CT3M has changed my life. By the beginning of 2012, I had been on synthetic T4-only medication for close to 11 years. I had gained 100 pounds and was depressed, anxious, suicidal, chronically fatigued, having reproductive issues, and more.

At that time, I struggled to get out of bed in the mornings. Once I did, I still struggled for about the next three hours to wake up. I would have a burst of energy for an hour or two, then crash.

Taking care of my children, showering, and eating were arduous tasks. Any sort of decision-making would send me into a tailspin. I was hardly able to leave the house, and if I did it would take me days to recover. Any sort of significant physical exertion was exhausting.

All of this affected my family as well, and I relied on my Mom to help me on a regular basis. My struggles gave my husband constant stress and worry. He was doing practically all the grocery shopping and meal preparations. I agonised over my inability to be the mother that I wanted to be. I longed to do the simple things, like take my young daughters to the library and play groups, craft, learn with them at home, and just enjoy each other's company without worrying how every little thing would affect me physically or mentally.

During the worst period of my health issues, I would lay in bed at night wondering if I were dying from a deadly disease - and yet I was petrified that I was not dying, and that this was the way I was going to be for the rest of my life.

I had heard about natural desiccated thyroid (NDT) and switched to that, but I always knew there was more to my problems than just hypothyroidism. I started learning about thyroid and adrenal dysfunction through the patient-to-patient organisation 'Stop the Thyroid Madness.'

It was through the STTM discussion groups that I met Paul Robinson, and learned about his book and the Circadian T3 Method (CT3M). I did a 24-hour cortisol saliva test, and discovered that I had low daytime cortisol with elevated nighttime levels. And so I began CT3M with my NDT.

Within a few weeks of starting the method, I noted that my fatigue was no longer extreme. Also, waking up in the mornings wasn't as much of a struggle and I wasn't pining for caffeine as much. My flu-like aches, afternoon 'slump', and chronic low back pain were improved. I was no longer taking days to recuperate from everyday little things like grocery shopping, or running a couple of errands with my young children.

I had less anxiety and depression, and my suicidal thoughts were gone. I was able to hold my children while standing up for longer periods of time. I was no longer easily winded. I started ovulating again and my endometriosis pain lessened. I started losing some excess weight. I also found that my feet were no longer itching, burning, and sore.

The changes I was experiencing were dramatic, but I was still far from well. After about 4-6 weeks of using CT3M, I began having trouble increasing my dose. I found out I had very low storage iron, which was preventing my body from properly converting the T4 in my NDT into T3.

With Paul's *Recovering with T3* book, and his observations on the experience of thyroid patients with CT3M, I decided to change my early morning dose to T3-only and to take my NDT in the afternoon. I knew that this would help provide me with the T3 I was lacking whilst I was raising my iron levels.

The second day of taking T3 for my circadian dose, my body temperature rose earlier in the day (closer to normal) and improved further by mid-afternoon. I was less irritable, had less dizziness, less nausea. My afternoon sleepiness hit me later in the afternoon.

After a few weeks of using T3 for my circadian dose, I found that I was able to raise my dose from 15 mcg of T3 to 18.75 mcg. I also raised my afternoon NDT dose from 1 grain to 1.5, and then later to 2 grains. This told me that my adrenals were healing, which meant my cortisol was rising and allowing more T3 to enter my cells as well.

In addition to using CT3M, I am also taking supplements, including: iron bis-glycinate, Vitamin C, Vitamin D3, magnesium, iodine, selenium, methyl-B12 and astaxanthin. I work hard to ensure that I get adequate sleep at night by going to bed and waking at the same time every day. I eliminated gluten from my diet, which gives me reactions identical to my old hypothyroid and adrenal fatigue symptoms. I focus on eating nutritious, non-processed foods. Finally, I have learned how to pace myself and listen attentively to my body.

Now I feel better than I have felt in years. I currently take 18.75 mcg T3 at 5:30 am (circadian dose); 1 grain NDT + 6.25 mcg T3 at 10 am; 1 grain at 2 pm; 6.25 mcg T3 at 5 pm. This regime is the solution I need to feel well.

I have no depression or anxiety. I'm losing weight, and I rise in the mornings with only a little effort. I can prepare meals, clean the house, care for and play with my children, run errands, and live life with much less caution and concern for how every little thing might affect my adrenals. I confidently look forward to more improvement with continued use of the method, listening to my body, good nutrition and quality sleep.

Paul's Observations: I think there are some strong similarities in Mary's story to that of Sue's. However, in Mary's case, she is more typical of the majority of thyroid patients who actually do need a near full replacement of thyroid hormone in order to feel well. Mary uses a combination of T3 for CT3M (the circadian dose), and a combination of NDT and T3 doses in the daytime. Let me make a few observations:

1. The range of symptoms associated with hypothyroidism that has induced partial adrenal insufficiency can be huge. These symptoms are often physical, but can also affect the brain and mental health well-being, e.g. 'brain fog', depression.

2. The type of thyroid medication (or combination) that best suits the thyroid patient cannot always be determined in advance, but has to be discovered by trying one type and finding out if it works well, or not. If the medication is not sufficiently effective, then another type of thyroid medication (or a combination) may be tried, often with great success. Mary began treating her hypothyroidism by using NDT for all her doses. She eventually had more success with T3 for the circadian dose, and NDT and T3 doses in the daytime. T4 was totally unhelpful for Mary, as it is for many thyroid patients.

3. Individual patients need individual solutions. When thyroid patients achieve these tailored solutions, they tend to get well in a way that can be astonishing. The transformation can be startling, wonderful and beautiful to watch.

4. Improvement in symptoms can occur very quickly once the right thyroid medication (or combination), and the suitable dosing strategy for the individual, is discovered.

5. Supplementation with appropriate nutrients can be hugely beneficial to support the healing process, and to help maintain good health.

6. As with Sue's story, a focus on overall health and diet can be extraordinarily important. The health of the gut, and the maintenance of gut integrity and gut flora balance, is crucial for many thyroid patients.

7. A major recovery from a wide range of debilitating symptoms is actually possible. Thyroid patients do not have to be imprisoned within their own bodies for the rest of their lives if the whole person/whole body is looked at and all issues are addressed.

Often, it needs the thyroid patient themselves to champion this, and to get their head down and get on with it. Taking responsibility for your own health can be the most important part of recovery.

JULIE'S STORY

I always considered the onset of my hypothyroid symptoms started just after the birth of my first child in 1986. I was 25 at the time. Looking back, however, I wonder if my teenage depression, mood swings, painful periods and severe PMT were early warning signs of things to come.

After the birth of my first child I was diagnosed with post-natal depression and anaemia, both of which continued throughout my next two pregnancies and beyond. I popped iron supplements like sugar pills, but never seemed to significantly raise my levels (no-one ever told me that iron should be taken with vitamin C to be properly absorbed).

Fatigue, depression and weight gain became consistent after my third child in 1991. I would fall asleep in the car whilst waiting outside the kid's school - slumped like a lardy, snoozing hippo in the driver's seat, and would park around the corner in the hope of grabbing 40 winks undetected by passing, more dynamic, mothers.

My doctor reassured me that this was all completely normal with three small children, and placated me with a 6-month course of anti-depressants. I gratefully accepted these in the hope of dropkicking myself out of the black hole I was steadily sinking into.

Despite continued dieting, I gained 4 stone over the next 15 years. This intensified my depression, and sent my self-confidence slithering away down the back of the sofa along with the growing evidence of my neglected housework.

My fatigue also worsened, and I would drag myself out of my bed in the mornings, motivated only by the anticipation of my return to it, and then calculating potential snooze opportunities around the bare necessities of child-care. I was completely unable to enjoy what should have been the most wonderful years at home with my young children. My fatigue, depression and severe mood swings ensured that nobody else was enjoying them either.

My 6-month course of antidepressants turned into 12 years of Prozac treatment. This kept me from murder and suicide, but added further to my rapidly accumulating list of symptoms.

In 2006, after 15 years of steady weight gain, chronic fatigue, depression, headaches, mood swings, brain fog, memory loss, swelling legs, sporadic constipation and IBS (to name but a few), and numerous trips to the doctor, I was finally diagnosed with hypothyroidism by a locum whilst I was suffering from 'carpal tunnel syndrome'.

Although my TSH reading was only 6, I felt so relieved that my suspicions were finally recognised. I persuaded the doctor to put me on levothyroxine straight away, as, at that stage, I believed that my chronic health issues would soon be behind me, and that I would be dancing on rooftops in my favourite red dress (3 sizes too small) in two shakes of a lamb's tail.

With high hopes, I started on 25 mcg of levothyroxine and after a couple of weeks felt that things were improving slightly. Unfortunately, by the third week, they nose-dived and I actually felt worse. My doctor retested my TSH, declaring that everything was "now normal", and that there was nothing more to do but keep calm and carry on taking the pills!

My lifeline came when my sister, a nutritional therapist, gave me a copy of Dr Barry Peatfield's original book, *The Great Thyroid Scandal and How to Survive it*, and a new day dawned. This was my turning point, empowering me with information about alternative treatments for hypothyroidism (particularly natural desiccated thyroid) and the inadequacies of the standard medical approach of treatment based on blood test results rather than patients' symptoms.

The book also gave me the confidence to be more proactive in my treatment, and I found a private doctor who would prescribe me 'Armour thyroid'. Again, I felt better at first, but then my symptoms returned. On suspecting adrenal issues, I introduced adrenal glandular supplements and within a couple of weeks I was up and running.

I chugged along on 2 grains of Armour and 600 mg glandulars for the next two years, smugly confident with my new and greatly improved health. I weaned myself off Prozac, and switched to 150 mg 5HTP (5-hydroxytryptophan – a naturally occurring amino acid that may help to raise serotonin and melatonin levels, and is used by some doctors as an anti-depressant). I then restarted my low carbohydrate diet with renewed vigor, and over the next few months lost 2 1/2 stone. I was on fire and felt like life was finally looking up.

During this period I continued to read everything I could find on hypothyroidism, and on gaining a more thorough understanding of the subject became intrigued about the possibilities of T3. I asked my doctor if I could try adding some T3 to my daily Armour dose as, although much improved, I still had some lingering symptoms.

I added 10 mcgs of T3 to my 2 grains of Armour, and within days I felt my energy levels rise. Unfortunately, when my next thyroid tests were taken, my T3 was above the normal range so my daffy doctor became nervous, and I dropped it!

In 2010 I started back in full time work, but unfortunately my private doc retired and, as I had no time to find another doctor, I resorted to NHS T4 again. Within the next 6 months, I reverted to zombie-land, falling asleep at 8 pm and experiencing panic attacks in the office. I resigned a year later, and settled back onto my sofa to start researching again.

I managed to obtain Armour on the Internet and decided I needed to gradually raise my dose. Finding that this made my symptoms worse, I tried cutting right back. I re-started 3 times, but each time on reaching 3 grains my hypo symptoms worsened and I was left feeling confused and very ill.

I decided that if my body was becoming thyrotoxic when I reached this higher dose, that I must be building up a backlog of un-utilised T4, or possibly reverse T3, which was blocking conversion of T4 to T3. If I couldn't properly convert T4 into the useable T3, then why not just take T3 and go straight to the sharp end?

My NHS doctor said she had never even heard of liothyronine, so I wasted no more time and managed to find a source myself. None of the books that had cursorily mentioned T3 gave any detail of its proper use or titration. So, I decided to check out patient forums for any mention of this illusive and now intriguing medication.

In the meantime, I stopped taking Armour for as long as I could stand (5 days). I started my new protocol on 1st July 2011, on one 1/2 tablet of T3 twice a day. On the fourth day I felt amazing and increasingly excited about this new life... and that red dress!

Unfortunately, my miraculous improvement started to wane slightly around week 4. I reintroduced the adrenal glandulars and decided to slowly raise the T3 in 3-4 divided doses. Within three months I was taking 25 mcg at 8 am, 25 mcg at 12.00 noon, 2 mcg at 5 pm and 18.75 mcg at bedtime, along with 1000 mg of Nutri Adrenal (an adrenal glandular).

However, I began to flounder at this point. My heart rate was sporadically high with occasional palpitations, and some mornings I just felt like crap. There was no real consistency. I felt gutted that I had tasted the other side of life, which was now slipping away from me. I couldn't judge whether my symptoms indicated over or under stimulation. I spent hours lying on my bed going over and over the facts in my foggy head, trying to analyse where I might be going wrong. I began to panic about what I had taken on.

When I found someone on a forum called 'puret3paul' (this ID is no longer in use) I realised that I had hit the jackpot! Paul Robinson was amazing, taking time to discuss my situation via email and sending me the manuscript of the book he was writing. I read his draft from cover to cover, and felt the ubiquitous light coming on, with renewed confidence in my chosen path. I was incredibly reassured by his knowledge and detailed research.

The Circadian T3 Method (CT3M) particularly intrigued me. I had already taken an adrenal test only a few weeks after starting T3, and it had been completely normal. As a result, I had slowly dropped the adrenal supplements and was on a daily total of 92.75 mcg T3 only. However, I'd only stopped the adrenal glandulars two days prior to the adrenal saliva test. I now realise that this was not enough time for them to be out of my body; I should have stopped them at least two to three weeks before taking the adrenal saliva test.

After talking with Paul, however, I decided to give CT3M a chance. I dropped my doses down to three, halved them and took the first dose of T3 at 5 am within the main cortisol production window. Then, I slowly re-raised the doses.

Within 3 weeks I had raised to only 62.5 mcg and achieved my true 'Eureka' moment. I felt amazing, and have continued to feel better than I have for the last 15 years. I now have the energy to exercise my dogs for an hour at a time, and I can join my friends on beach walks rather than looking on from the coffee bar. I am continuing to lose weight because dieting actually works now, and my self-esteem has properly emerged from the sofa.

Over the last 18 months I have hit the menopause and suffered sleep disruption. After tweaking the CT3M dose and timings, I have found that adding an extra ¼ tablet has been most effective, which brings my daily regime to 25 mcg T3 at 5 am (circadian dose), 25 mcg at 11.30 am, 18.75 mcg at 4pm. This, along with a strict gluten free, low carb diet and good quality nutritional supplements has kept me happy, healthy and full of determination to find a new red dress.

I bought Paul Robinson's printed book *Recovering with T3,* as soon as it came out, and it will always hold a special place in my heart and on the bookshelf. I would urge anyone who has any interest in taking responsibility for their own health and recovery to do the same - simply the most important book I have ever read in my life! Good luck!

Paul's Observations: Julie's story is somewhat typical of thyroid patients who use T3 and CT3M:

1. It can take a long time for thyroid issues to be properly tested, and then diagnosed. This is a great shame and a major flaw in many healthcare systems. I think it goes right to the heart of medical training, not giving enough time to the diagnosis and proper treatment of thyroid disease. Thyroid disease is fairly easy to diagnose if the full range of laboratory tests are run at an early stage (TSH, FT4, FT3, reverse T3, TPO and Tg autoantibodies). In addition, sufficient attention needs to be given to the entire range of the patient's symptoms and signs. Often, symptoms are treated as being discrete issues, and the overall condition of the patient is not looked at. A simple trial with NDT or NDT/T3, or even T3 only, might be all that is required to confirm the diagnosis. Off my soapbox!

2. The range of symptoms of thyroid disease is often wide, especially when partial adrenal insufficiency is present too. It can take years for a proper diagnosis, and by that time the individual may have been on anti-depressants and have far more health issues that have occurred as a consequence of the thyroid problems. The impact on someone's life, and the people they are close to, can be profound.

3. Levothyroxine (T4) works for some thyroid patients, but leaves many with symptoms of hypothyroidism that often get far worse over time as adrenal issues develop. Levothyroxine is a poor choice, and ideally the T4 should be swapped for natural desiccated thyroid or T3. A T4/T3 combination might also be considered, but I really have little confidence in levothyroxine these days, as I've seen the havoc it can cause.

4. Information is power: gaining knowledge fast is often the best strategy. Consequently, books such as *Recovering with T3, Stop the Thyroid Madness, Your Thyroid and How to Keep it Healthy,* and others are hugely important to read to bootstrap this knowledge acquisition as fast as possible. Joining patient forums is also a great way to learn.

5. Finding a doctor (or doctors) you can work and discuss things with is also a great help. This can take time, and a few changes of doctor may be needed until someone that is

empathetic to the thyroid patient is found. However, this is also a key strategy and the effort is worth it.

6. Julie's daily T3 dosage at almost 70mcg is fairly typical of T3 users. Of course there are variations, with some thyroid patients taking higher levels than this, and some less. This is a more typical dosage as compared with Sue's, whose major health issue was related to partial adrenal insufficiency.

7. Nutritional supplements (including vitamins and minerals), and dietary changes to exclude irritants such as gluten, are another common theme in successful recovery from thyroid disease. These also enabled Julie to return from debilitating symptoms to great health.

8. Things change over time, and sometimes new issues emerge which need addressing. In Julie's case, the onset of the menopause required her to need to further adjust her thyroid medication. Others may need to consider the use of bio-identical sex hormones, or different supplements, or address other issues.

DEREK'S STORY

I was diagnosed as hypothyroid in June 2010. At the time my TSH was 7.6 ulU/mL, FT4 11.64pmol/L and FT3 5.29pmol/L. I was prescribed levothyroxine at a starting dose of 50 mcg. Initially I improved, and I also lost a bit of weight from the 105kg which I'd reached. My asthma and rhinitis also disappeared.

However, 3 months later I started to put on weight again, and I began to experience joint pain. I found out about Liothyronine (T3), and was fortunate to find a GP who would prescribe it. I then began to take T4 at 50 mcg and T3 at 20 mcg. Yet again initially I improved; however a month later all my symptoms reappeared. So I persuaded my GP to allow me to stop taking T4 completely and to increase my T3 dosage to 40 mcg. For another month I was fine, and then the pain symptoms returned, so my T3 dose was increased to 80mcg. I started to lose weight and reached 78kg, yet I still did not have the energy to exercise.

Then I bought the book *Recovering with T3*. As a consequence, I adjusted the way I took my T3 tablets - instead of taking T3 all in one dose, I split this as follows: 20 mcg at 5:00 am (CT3M dose), 20 mcg at 11.00 am, 20 mcg at 3:00 pm, 20 mcg at 7:00 pm. As a result, my pulse steadied and my blood pressure returned to normal.

2 1/2 years later, I have fine-tuned the method due to changing to a Paleo diet. I started experiencing shakes, so I realised that I was over-stimulated. I reduced my total 80mcg daily dose by 20mcg down to 60mcg. I also changed the dosage times too, and reduced the 4 doses down to 3. The times of my current doses are: circadian dose at 5:00 am, 12:00 noon then 5:00 pm.

I now have far more energy, and my weight is stable at 77kg. I'm enjoying cycling long distances. I do take vitamins and minerals, and I currently have no symptoms.

Paul's Observations: Derek's story is very typical of a thyroid patient who really needs T3 medication as his main treatment, but finds that his partial adrenal insufficiency requires CT3M also to correct it:

1. Levothyroxine (T4) was a poor treatment for Derek. He would still be ill today if he had remained on it. His symptoms would return within weeks if he went back on to T4.

2. Three or four doses per day of T3 are often required when using T3 only.

3. It is often better to optimise the daytime thyroid medication as much as possible initially, introducing CT3M at a later stage if the symptoms of partial adrenal insufficiency are not too extreme. When they are extreme, CT3M can be started at the same time as first using a new thyroid medication, such as NDT or T3.

4. Derek's experience suggests, once again, that excellent health can be achieved if the right thyroid medication is selected for the individual, it is dosed in the most suitable way for them, and there is a focus on diet and other aspects of health.

NATALIA'S STORY

I used CT3M to wean myself off Hydrocortisone. Before starting HC I had most of the symptoms of low adrenal and low thyroid function, with thyroid lab results at the bottom of the normal range, and ferritin below range. The symptoms that were hardest to cope with were: anxiety, hypoglycemic episodes, an inability to sleep either at night or during the day, extreme anger and irritability, difficulty concentrating, increased pulse rate, air hunger, a very slow pulse rate and heart palpitations, and constant fatigue. My adrenal issues arose due to a series of infections, bad sleeping habits and not taking a good supplementation of vitamins and minerals.

During my 8 months on HC, I tried to increase my iron levels (and levels of other vitamins), hoping that my low thyroid symptoms would disappear with enough cortisol and iron.

In November 2012, I decided to wean myself off HC. I had previously never taken any thyroid hormones. CT3M worked fantastically well in helping me to wean off HC. I used 10-12 mcg of T3 3-4 hours before getting up, and for the first few days I moved the first dose of HC to a later time and completely dropped the last HC dose. Every few days, I decreased the size of each HC dose, moving the first dose a little later in time and then dropping the then last (latest in time) HC dose. The final HC dose, which I dropped, was the middle day dose of 7 mg taken at 2 pm. This process was all completed in less than 3 weeks!

Amazingly, during those 3 weeks I did not feel any symptoms of low cortisol. During that time I had to add several T3 doses during the day (each no more then 12 mcg). I continued to stay on T3 only medication and CT3M for 3 more weeks, and I did not experience any low adrenal symptoms. I did, however, have some minor headaches appearing and disappearing during the day, which I believe were related to imbalanced levels of thyroid hormones, as I was not very consistent with my T3 dosing!

Then I weaned myself off T3 too. When I stopped using T3 as a circadian dose, I immediately noticed some symptoms of low cortisol, but they were tolerable. I had slight occasional dizziness, weakness and an inability to exercise or walk uphill. But these symptoms reduced, and I started feeling better and better every day.

Now, 5 months later, I feel pretty good during the day. All those symptoms are gone. I am still amazed that I now have the energy to wash dishes in the evening, or to brush my children's teeth. I can sleep now, too. CT3M was an amazing help in weaning off HC. My thyroid levels are ok now, due to both improved cortisol and iron levels. Thank you CT3M!

Paul's Observations: Natalia's story is quite unusual, in that she used CT3M as support to wean off adrenal steroids only. I don't have many observations on this as Natalia has explained things so clearly:

1. Natalia had partial adrenal insufficiency only. She was not taking any type of thyroid medication at all, and any symptoms of hypothyroidism were believed to be due to low cortisol, low iron levels or other low nutrients like B vitamins.

2. The adrenal steroid hydrocortisone (HC) was being used simply to provide the extra cortisol that Natalia needed in order to cope.

3. Natalia followed the process that many thyroid patients have found to be effective when weaning HC. She pushed the first dose of HC later in time, so that it was no longer within a few hours of the circadian dose. This means that the adrenals have time to work and respond to CT3M without a dose of HC arriving and suppressing them again (due to a lowering of ACTH). At the same time, she moved all other HC doses later in time, and weaned the last HC dose completely. Chapter 19 of this book covers the experience of thyroid patients when weaning steroids.

4. Adrenal steroids may be weaned within a few weeks. It is often better to do this quite quickly and replace with CT3M so that the process does not drag on for months. **This process should only be attempted in cases of partial adrenal insufficiency of course. Those with diseases like Addison's disease, or hypopituitarism, or other conditions that need long-term steroid use, will not be able to wean adrenal steroids**.

5. Correcting iron levels and other nutrients must have been a huge factor in Natalia's recovery, as she was then able to stop using T3 and CT3M. This again emphasises how important diet, nutrient intake and gut health are for all of us.

CHRISTEL'S STORY

I started CT3M a year after my full thyroidectomy (2010). The year before I had tried everything: T4, NDT, the 'old school' T3 only protocol to clear RT3. Nothing helped - I felt better, but not at all anywhere near optimal.

I supported my weak adrenals with Isocort (an adrenal glandular) and even HC for a short while, which I did not tolerate at all. So I just stopped taking HC, as I felt it made me sicker. After reaching a total dose of 100mcg T3, and my hypo symptoms returning with a vengeance, I was at a loss about what to do next.

It was at that point that I stumbled upon a post on a thyroid forum about CT3M. This was just a month or so before the *Recovering with T3* book came out. With help from the posts, which Paul had put on that forum, and from other people who were also using CT3M, I thought I'd try it (since I saw no other way), and it helped. Immediately, the worst of my symptoms lessened. As I progressed and found my sweet spot for the circadian dose in terms of timing and dosage size, I felt at 80% of my total health. Of course, by then, I had ordered and read the book, and I knew I had some more obstacles to overcome.

During the summer of 2012 (after a stressful week with almost no decent sleep), I felt horrible again. I had some blood tests carried out, and my iron levels were very low. So I learnt that I had to keep taking iron supplementation, as my levels will not stay high without a maintenance dose. I also found out that I had some blood sugar issues, which are now under control. But I still felt that after 'the crash' there was something 'off', so I took a saliva test. The saliva test showed morning cortisol to be at the top of the range, both noon and evening cortisol levels to be low, and nighttime level at mid-range.

I decided to take my circadian dose much later. This led to another lesson being learned; namely in my case, that my adrenals will always need to be supported by CT3M dosing, and I cannot make jumps in circadian dose timing that are too large.

So now I feel much better again, and I guess the last hurdle will be increasing my progesterone levels, as I am nearing menopausal years. I have recently doubled my dose, and will do so for a month or two and see what happens. I already notice I feel less sweaty and less tired.

I now take a total of 62.5 mcg of T3 in 3 divided doses. My CT3M dose is 25 mcg, taken at 5.30 am, which is a time that I sometimes tweak depending on my stress levels. I am still learning, but I have gotten my life back. I know I'll have to deal with some 'off' days once in a while, and I just go with the flow when that happens. It is a long and meticulous journey, but for me CT3M is working. I just know I will always need to be vigilant and flexible in adjusting timing according to how I am feeling.

Paul's Observations: Christel's story is quite typical of many thyroid patients:

1. So many people that have used adrenal steroids (such as HC) and adrenal glandulars have said to me that they just do not feel well on them. Regardless of the dosing of these steroids, or what thyroid medication is being used with them, many thyroid patients never feel well on them. Clearly, some people absolutely do need adrenal

steroids, but many thyroid patients have been persuaded to try them without the necessary medical diagnosis that supports their use e.g. real Addison's disease, hypopituitarism or a condition that requires steroids as part of its treatment.

2. Christel's response to CT3M is also very typical. CT3M tends to enable the adrenal glands to work more effectively during the day. This is quite different from the peaks and troughs of adrenal hormone levels that result when one or two adrenal hormones have been taken from a bottle.

3. As with most people, thyroid hormone balance and CT3M are only one part of the solution. There has to be a focus on the entire person, and on dealing with other problems if they exist. In Christel's case, she mentions blood sugar issues and sex-hormone balance (presumably to correct oestrogen dominance, which is often a problem for peri-menopausal women).

4. Some people will eventually be able to wean themselves off CT3M and no longer use a circadian dose. Others like Christel, and myself, will always need it due to some change that occurred in the body after the onset of thyroid disease and partial adrenal insufficiency. I do not know whether this change is due to an alteration in the HPA axis, or due to the adrenals themselves, or simply due to the fact that taking thyroid medication is just not the same as having it manufactured on demand by your own thyroid in response to TSH. I suspect it is more the latter, but this is hard to prove without access to medical research to investigate this.

5. Situations change over time. Menopause is an example of a large change. However, smaller factors like a change in the amount of stress we are under, or the level of activity we are involved in, may be enough to create a need for an adjustment in thyroid medication dosage, CT3M dose size/timing or some other hormone.

HELEN'S STORY

I had increasingly high cortisol levels over a 5-year period. Then, in 2010, my cortisol levels dropped to below normal, the morning level being the lowest point of the day. In 2012 I discovered Paul Robinson's CT3M method of improving cortisol, and I started using that approach in July. I didn't notice a lot of difference during the first couple of months, and my saliva cortisol test results were still low. However, Paul pointed out that if I had blood sugar issues, CT3M would not work properly. So I took both fasting and non-fasting blood tests, which showed that I did have blood sugar issue problems. I'd heard about Metformin, a prescription drug used for insulin resistance, so I asked my doctor if I would be able to try it. Since then, I've had several tests that seem to confirm that I have insulin resistance.

I started taking Metformin in late October, and continued with the CT3M dose and time that seemed to work best for me, being 20 mcg of T3 three hours before getting up. By early

December, my cortisol levels had improved and were back to normal, and my morning cortisol was even just over the normal level range! So once I had my blood sugar in check, CT3M worked really quickly for me.

Since tapering off my circadian dose, I have noticed that I need less T3 for my thyroid dosing, which is exciting. My head is becoming clearer, and I am feeling so much better than I did. I do take things gradually, as I don't want to revert back to low cortisol again, and I think I'm getting stronger by the day.

I am currently working on finding a low, or late in the window (of cortisol production), circadian dose that works as a maintenance dose. I am so grateful to Paul for the huge amount of time and energy he has spent researching and testing to discover something that is bringing relief to so many of us.

Paul's Observations: Helen's story illustrates once again that CT3M is not a solution in its own right that will fix adrenal health, but something that can be immensely helpful when combined with the treatment of other important issues:

1. Helen did not get much of a response at all to CT3M when she first used it. It required the discovery of the health issue that was holding her back before CT3M would work. In Helen's case, it was a blood sugar problem, in that her insulin was not allowing glucose to enter her cells in sufficient volume. As such, Helen's cells would not have been able to make sufficient energy (ATP) to support thyroid hormone action.

2. Once the insulin resistance had been diagnosed and treated, Helen responded well to CT3M.

3. The trick now is that Helen really doesn't need a great deal of CT3M support, but she may need a minor maintenance dose of CT3M. This requires some fine-tuning, and may require very subtle changes in the timing of the circadian dose or the dose size. It is hard to predict which will work best. Simply picking a dose size and moving it later in time (and seeing if there is a point it begins to be ideal) is the way to do it.

4. During this type of fine-tuning of a maintenance CT3M dose, some people can achieve benefits from a timing that is 1.5 hours before get-up time, and some can take it later, i.e. closer to the get-up time. During fine-tuning, 30 minute, 15 minute, or even 10 minute adjustments can be helpful. Size adjustments of the order of 5 micrograms of T3, or 2.5 micrograms of T3, can also be helpful.

FRANCIS'S STORY

I am currently 32 years old and have the following conditions: PCOS, Addison's disease, Hashimoto's, interstitial cystitis and coeliac disease.

I have had adrenal insufficiency symptoms ever since I can remember. As a child I always felt faint when I stood up (classic postural hypotension), I craved salt, I had an anxious personality and I had sleep problems. I actually had adrenal symptoms long before I developed thyroid symptoms. My thyroid symptoms first appeared at the age of 16.

When I was 14, I suffered second-degree burns to my thighs and hips, and had to spend a month in a burns unit. I believe that this is what triggered a cascade of endocrine dysfunction, and I am sure it was yet another blow to my already under functioning adrenal system. At that age, I also began vomiting every morning. This was not done purposely; I simply developed extreme nausea in the mornings. I hated school at the time, so the doctor put it down to that. I now know that nausea and/or vomiting in the mornings is a classic adrenal symptom.

At the age of 16, I developed severe depression completely out of the blue for no reason at all. I began seeing a variety of psychiatrists from the age of 16 to 25. I have nothing but praise for how lovely they were to me. In fact, I would go so far as to say that the psychiatrists I saw were the kindest group of specialists I've ever encountered, unlike the horrible endocrinologists I've dealt with in my time! However, it never occurred to them to check my thyroid or adrenal function.

From the age of 16 to 28 I suffered the usual thyroid and adrenal symptoms: heavy and extremely painful periods, severe depressions that would appear out of nowhere and leave me suicidal, dry skin, stomach problems, plantar fasciitis, severe coldness, high cholesterol and weight gain. I also always had the aforementioned adrenal symptoms. The weight gain caused me to develop an eating disorder that nearly killed me. Ironically, the eating disorder did not even result in any type of sustained weight loss. It just caused misery.

Eventually, at the age of 28, I went to see a trainee psychiatrist who told me that my symptoms sounded like classic hypothyroidism. He told me that I needed to be tested. I went to see my GP, who pronounced me normal since I had a TSH of 1.64 and a FT4 of 15 (12-22). I really felt in my bones that I had hypothyroidism, and actually felt sad when she told me that I didn't. She also told me, "Everyone who comes in here thinks they have a thyroid problem".

A few months later, I googled "doctors" and found one who specialised in diagnosing unexplained illnesses. I made an appointment with him, and he sent me for comprehensive tests. I took a saliva cortisol test, which showed my total cortisol was below range: the only time it barely crept into the normal range was at night. I also had my FT3 and antibodies tested. My antibodies were very high, and my FT3 was only 0.1 away from the bottom of the range. He put me on adrenal glandulars, but sadly did not do an ACTH stimulation test.

After a few months he told me that my adrenals would now be strong enough to cope with thyroid hormone. So I started on 1/4 grain of natural thyroid. I then moved up to 1/2 a grain. Unfortunately, my low cortisol then reared its head and I developed debilitating palpitations, heart pounding and extreme anxiety. I went back to the doctor who then told me that this meant I needed hydrocortisone. I started on hydrocortisone in early 2008. I have never been able to come off it.

I eventually stopped seeing this doctor, as he would not raise my natural thyroid. I tried some other doctors, but had no joy. After a while, the natural thyroid stopped working, and most of my thyroid symptoms came back.

After a lot of reading, I realised in 2010 that I needed T3 only. However, no doctor would prescribe me T3 only. So I self treated, which was a complete and utter disaster. I did not have Paul's book at the time, so I started on too high a dose and increased it too quickly. As a result, it went very wrong and I had to go back to natural thyroid.

Eventually, in late 2011, I found an excellent doctor who knew all about thyroid resistance. He was concerned that I had only ever had an adrenal saliva test. He felt that I did indeed have adrenal insufficiency that would require lifelong HC treatment; however he also wanted to do some further testing. So I was admitted to hospital and had a 24-hour urine screen, and morning and afternoon serum testing. Naturally, my cortisol was low at all times. Therefore, **I was officially diagnosed with Addison's disease** and my GP is now happy to continue to prescribe me HC. My consultant suspects that I have a form of LOCAH (Late Onset Congenital Adrenal Hyperplasia), which is a type of adrenal disorder that presents with symptoms similar to PCOS. However, there is no accurate test for this whilst on steroids, so for now my diagnosis is Addison's disease. This doctor also started me on T3 only in February 2012, by which time I had read the *Recovering with T3* book.

Thanks to HC, I was able to tolerate sufficient T3 only to get rid of my thyroid symptoms. Despite being warned that I would need more HC in order to tolerate T3 only, this did not happen. I feel amazing on T3 only. Family members even commented that T3 was like "rocket fuel", and that I was back to my old self within two months of taking T3 only.

In 2012, **I also started CT3M. Even though I take hydrocortisone**, I find that CT3M makes all the difference when it comes to my sleep disorder. I take 40 mcg of T3 and 10 mg of HC at 7.30 am and get up between 8.30 am - 9.00 am. For the first time in my life, I am now able to rise at this time without feeling like someone is shaking me from a coma. Up until this combination of T3 and HC for the CT3M dose, I was only able to get up at 10 am at the earliest, and I usually rose at 11 a.m.

I then take 40 mcg of T3 and 10 mg of HC at noon, and my final dose is 40 mcg of T3 and 5 mg HC at 5 pm.

I did try CT3M without the use of steroids, but unfortunately my low cortisol symptoms returned with a vengeance: shaking, hypoglycaemia, anxiety, heart palpitations and postural hypotension.

The combination of T3 and HC together in CT3M seems to make all the difference to me. I may tweak it again in the future to see if I can rise earlier by taking it earlier, as I still cannot function if I get up before 8 am. If I rise before this time I spend the day with postural hypotension, extreme nausea and shakiness. However, for now it has given me a much better quality of life. I can actually start my day's work at 9 am. like a normal person now, and can schedule activities in the morning. This has never been possible throughout my entire life.

After much thought, I have now come to the conclusion that patients with Addison's disease have some adrenal function remaining. Some have more than others. There is a range of remaining adrenal function. Some do not have enough for any quality of life, and eventually the adrenals will go kaput completely and a person may die, but it takes decades to get there generally. Therefore, I feel the reason that I responded to CT3M is that my adrenals are kind of like a broken car that splutters and stops. I have a small degree of adrenal function left, which may be why it works for me. Other patients may be in the same situation.

The combination of T3 only and CT3M have been miraculous. It is like a light switch has been turned on. My life would be completely different without both of them.

Paul's Observations: Francis's story shows another creative way CT3M is being used by thyroid patients:

1. I never believed that CT3M could be used in combination with HC use, but here is one thyroid patient that is doing so successfully, and it is allowing her to live her life.

2. I have also stated that it is unlikely that CT3M can help a patient who has an Addison's disease diagnosis, but real life has also proven me wrong! I am actually very happy for this patient that this is the case. I have every expectation that I will be surprised again by the creativity that thyroid patients often have when they are trying to get well.

3. This story also illustrates how (for some patients) the use of T3 appears to be a big benefit when implementing CT3M.

LESSONS

There are two lessons that I took away from the above thyroid patient stories.

Firstly, CT3M can be a very useful tool in the effort to restore adrenal function and is often far superior to adrenal steroids and adrenal glandulars.

Secondly, CT3M is only one strategy to employ. Very often one or more other problems need to be identified and then resolved. Diet, gut health and appropriate nutrient supplementation often have as critical a role in the recovery of adrenal health as CT3M. In some cases, specific issues with sex hormones, methylation issues, inflammation, toxicity or immune system imbalances will need to be resolved. If there are any underlying chronic health issues, then they may well need to be identified and addressed (see Chapter 8 for some of these).

CT3M is a simple and helpful tool in the restoration of healthy adrenal function, but it is just one tool. For some it will be the only tool needed. For others, CT3M will be one of many tools, and for some it may not be relevant or very helpful at all.

Chapter 23

Final Comments

When I first wrote *Recovering with T3*, I had no idea that one part of my T3 dosage management process, called the Circadian T3 Method (CT3M), would:

- Be effective with either T3 or NDT medication.
- Support the use of combinations of thyroid medication i.e. with NDT or T3 for the circadian dose, followed by NDT or T3 daytime thyroid doses.
- Be powerful to so many thyroid patients suffering with partial adrenal insufficiency.
- Be effective enough to allow thyroid patients to wean themselves (within a few weeks) from the use of adrenal steroids or glandulars, and simply use CT3M.
- Be valuable to thyroid patients who have partial adrenal insufficiency (but only very minor thyroid hormone issues).
- Be valuable alongside HC, for those thyroid patients that have severe partial adrenal insufficiency, or an Addison's disease diagnosis.

It is now apparent that CT3M is a valuable approach, and one that will continue to be used for many years to come. Hopefully, over time, the medical profession will become increasingly aware of the potential of this relatively simple and natural approach to improving the adrenal function of those thyroid patients for whom this is applicable.

FOR THOSE ABOUT TO BEGIN USING CT3M

The following four points are important to note for those starting out using CT3M:

1. The thyroid patients who have the smoothest, most effective and rapid response with CT3M often already have a good diet, are taking a wide range of vitamin and mineral supplements, and have good iron levels. They tend also to have addressed other health issues before starting CT3M.

2. For someone who is trying to lower reverse T3 (rT3) by switching from levothyroxine (T4) to either NDT or T3, it may take a considerable amount of time before rT3 actually reduces and clears (typically 8-12 weeks). During this period, CT3M may not be as effective, and patience will be needed until the rT3 has cleared.

3. Weaning adrenal steroids quite quickly is often an effective strategy. This clearly needs to be done with the support of a knowledgeable doctor, and in a controlled way that is well monitored. However, thyroid patients have often found that they feel better once they do begin to wean these steroids. Steroids can always be added back if a negative impact from weaning is discovered.

4. **Some thyroid patients cannot under any circumstances wean adrenal steroids. Any thoughts about weaning adrenal steroids should be discussed with the patient's own medical physician.**

Patience is crucial when applying CT3M. Sufficient time should be allowed to watch and analyse the response to a circadian dose change. It is counter-productive to raise the dose or change the timing too quickly, and without gathering enough information. Lack of patience may introduce poor choices, and this can result in the frequent need to re-start CT3M all over again.

For a thyroid patient with partial adrenal insufficiency, CT3M is a safe, simple approach, which is well worth trying before using adrenal steroids or adrenal glandulars.

CT3M should be the first choice treatment in these situations, and it may help many thyroid patients to avoid ever having to use adrenal steroids. For those thyroid patients already using adrenal glandulars or adrenal steroids, CT3M may be able to offer improved health and the prospect of weaning these drugs.

MEDICAL PROFESSION RESPONSE TO CT3M SO FAR

The response from doctors has been slightly better than I expected. I have received dozens of reports from thyroid patients that their doctor is happy to work with them in using CT3M as part of their treatment program. Most of these open-minded doctors appear to be from the USA, but a few are from the UK, Europe and elsewhere.

A typical response from an endocrinologist or doctor is that they have not heard of CT3M, would not read the book and that it won't work. Of course, most of these aren't even aware of the latest research on the circadian pattern of FT3, and some may not even know about the circadian nature of cortisol production (which has been known about for decades). This response is as I expected. If something isn't taught in medical school, and it has not been communicated by another doctor, or through a medical journal, then it is likely to be written off as nonsense. Few doctors look to patients for information.

The majority of doctors that have been made aware of CT3M by a patient have simply dismissed it with a comment like, "This won't work!" This type of response is often quick, has not involved reading the *Recovering with T3* book, and has not included any practical experience or evaluation of CT3M. It is a shame, but it is also entirely predictable.

Many endocrinologists and doctors do not even believe that some of their patients have adrenal issues, especially if a Synacthen test has been passed, or there has been a cortisol blood test that has a result anywhere within the reference range!

Consequently, there is no surprise that many doctors, who hear about CT3M from patients, quickly discount it. CT3M exists to help improve adrenal function in the case of partial adrenal insufficiency. If a thyroid patient goes into their doctor's office clutching the *Recovering with T3* book, or this handbook, they should not be surprised to be told that, "CT3M is nonsense", or that, "it won't work!" There should be no surprise if a doctor tells their patient that T3 or NDT are not required, and that taking levothyroxine (T4) is all that is required for them to be healthy! It is a predictable response.

We now know that CT3M helps many thyroid patients with partial adrenal insufficiency. It may not work for all, as some issues appear to make it much harder for CT3M to work well. However, we are continuously increasing our learning about the issues that prevent an optimal response to CT3M. I am, therefore, highly optimistic that we will find more ways of dealing with these over time. I also sincerely hope that many more doctors will become open-minded and consider supporting their patients who wish to try CT3M.

WHY DO WE NEED THYROID MEDICATIONS THAT CONTAIN T3 AT ALL?

This is a question I have considered for many years. The incidence of patients who require either T3 or NDT appears to be increasing. Is there a reason for this? Dr. Sarah Myhill believes that many modern ailments result from either micro-nutrient deficiencies or toxic stress. I am absolutely sure that she is correct, and that this is a huge factor for many thyroid patients. An informative example is type 2 diabetes. A study published in *The Lancet* looked at the level of persistent organic pollutants in the normal population. What they found was that those with the highest level of pollutants, compared to the lowest level, were 38 times more likely to be diabetic. It is recognised that type 2 diabetes is not due to insulin deficiencies, but to insulin resistance – that is to say the insulin receptor is blocked.

I believe we are seeing a similar situation with thyroid hormones. The fact that often supra-physiological doses of T3 have to be used to get a clinical result tells us that there is thyroid hormone receptor resistance in many of these patients. It is biologically plausible that this hormone receptor resistance results from toxins in the environment, and indeed the recently published *Oxford Textbook of Endocrinology and Diabetes* lists ways in which toxins interfere with thyroid hormone production and hormone receptor blockage.

What this means is that detoxification regimes to identify these persistent organic pollutants, and get rid of them, may well be an important part of treatment of thyroid patients in the future. My focus in *Recovering with T3* and in this book has been to provide innovative treatment protocols that can work to overcome a range of issues. In the future, it may be possible to identify the root cause of the problem and deal with it directly.

FINALLY

Many thyroid patients have found that CT3M is a benefit to them in overcoming the symptoms of partial adrenal insufficiency. I remain positive in hoping that armed with the information within this book, more thyroid patients (working with their doctors), may be successful in using CT3M.

However, sometimes CT3M is not enough on its own to completely resolve all problems, and in some cases it may not work at all. CT3M is one of many tools available in the struggle to improve adrenal health in thyroid patients. It is very clear that the overall health of the thyroid patient has to be addressed, and this should include the investigation and treatment of any other health issues that may be present. Some of these underlying health issues may have no obvious unique symptoms, and the thyroid patient may have no idea that these issues are indeed present. However, many underlying health problems can actually impact the action of thyroid hormone and adrenal health and be stopping thyroid patients from getting well.

I am hopeful that in time, most of the conditions and situations that can undermine thyroid hormone action and CT3M will have more straightforward diagnostic and treatable approaches, thus enabling those people who really struggle to overcome partial adrenal insufficiency to actually do so.

CT3M attempts to mimic the way the body raises biologically active T3 levels (FT3) in the cells during the night, to coincide with the time that the adrenal glands produce high volumes of cortisol. The standard methods of providing T4, T4/T3, T3 or NDT medications do not mimic this natural physiological circadian process. CT3M addresses this issue, and can be a great asset for those thyroid patients who have adrenal issues.

Far from being a strange concept, CT3M is actually far closer to a physiological replacement of T3 than any other method of dosing thyroid hormone has ever managed to achieve until now.

I believe that CT3M should be the first choice treatment for partial adrenal insufficiency, especially when combined with a more comprehensive health improvement programme. I hope that over time more doctors within the medical profession will begin to see the merit in CT3M, and the value of thyroid medications such as NDT and T3.

In the future I expect to see drug delivery systems that can deliver individually tailored doses of T3 and/or T4 at specific times of the day and night. CT3M will be built into these systems. Beyond that I have a vision of thyroid medication systems that provide each individual with automatic real-time FT3 and FT4 measurement, combined with medication delivery to create perfect individually tailored profiles of thyroid hormones over twenty-four hours for thyroid patients. I may not see most of this but I believe it will come and I believe that the concept behind CT3M will be integrated into such future thyroid medication systems.

SECTION 4

APPENDICES & INDEX

Appendix A

Books for Further Reading

Paul Robinson: *Recovering with T3 My Journey from Hypothyroidism to Good Health Using the T3 Thyroid Hormone*. Elephant in the Room Books. Revised Edition 2013. ISBN 978-0-9570993-1-9.

Dr. John C. Lowe: *The Metabolic Treatment of Fibromyalgia*. Boulder, McDowell Publishing Company, 2000. ISBN 0-914609-02-05.

Janie A. Bowthorpe, M.Ed.: *Stop The Thyroid Madness. A Patient Revolution Against Decades of Inferior Thyroid Treatment*. Colorado, Laughing Grape Publishing, 2008. ISBN 978-0615-477121.

Datis Kharrazian: *Why Do I Still Have Thyroid Symptoms? When My Lab Tests Are Normal*. New York, Morgan James Publishing, 2010. ISBN 978-1-60037-670-2.

Dr. Natasha Campbell-McBride: *Gut and Psychology Syndrome: Natural Treatment for Autism, ADD/ADHD, Dyslexia, Dyspraxia, Depression, Schizophrenia...* MedInform Publishing. 2010. ISBN 978-0954852023.

William Davis, MD: *Wheat Belly*. Rodale. 2011. ISBN 978-1609611545.

Diane Sanfilippo: *Practical Paleo: A Customized Approach to Health and Whole-Foods Lifestyle*. Victory Belt Publishing. 2009. ISBN 978-1936608751.

Appendix B

Useful Websites

Recovering With T3 Website: http://recoveringwitht3.com or http://rwt3.com
- The purpose of recoveringwitht3.com is to provide information for people who are trying to recover from hypothyroidism using the T3 thyroid hormone.

Specific blog posts that discuss CT3M:
   http://recoveringwitht3.com/blog/what-circadian-t3-method
   http://recoveringwitht3.com/blog/why-circadian-t3-method-so-important
   http://recoveringwitht3.com/blog/background-circadian-t3-method-ct3m
   http://recoveringwitht3.com/blog/why-both-time-and-dose-size-adjustments-need-be-
      done-circadian-t3-method-ct3m
   http://recoveringwitht3.com/blog/circadian-t3-method-ct3m
   http://recoveringwitht3.com/blog/circadian-t3-method-supports-adrenal-glands-and-does-
      not-stress-them
   http://recoveringwitht3.com/blog/circadian-t3-method-and-weaning-adrenal-steroids
   http://recoveringwitht3.com/blog/more-circadian-dose-size-and-timing-adjustments
   http://recoveringwitht3.com/blog/interpretation-signs-ct3m-hr-bp-temp
   http://recoveringwitht3.com/blog/some-clarifications-circadian-t3-method-ct3m

Success stories with CT3M that have been submitted to the Recovering with T3 website may be viewed by clicking *circadian T3 method* on the menu on the right hand side of this page:
   http://recoveringwitht3.com/success_story

Recovering with T3 Facebook Page: http://www.facebook.com/recoveringwitht3
- Provides information regarding new updates to the Recovering with T3 website and additional information for people trying to recover from hypothyroidism using the T3 thyroid hormone.

Audio Recordings about CT3M

- There are three 10-minute audio recordings that explain how CT3M was developed and why it should be in the toolkit of thyroid patients and doctors:

    Part 1: http://www.youtube.com/watch?v=97SOyEYwh54.

    Part 2: http://www.youtube.com/watch?v=7t2wg9rr6F4.

    Part 3: http://www.youtube.com/watch?v=dhkhcLPGCww

Videos about CT3M

- There are three short video clips that explain how CT3M is applied:

    Part 1: http://youtu.be/YDV1qePLtLs

    Part 2: http://youtu.be/o-ye4Ci-EFw

    Part 3: http://youtu.be/dQ2QhW4H4ew

Thyroid Patient Advocacy Website: http://tpauk.com

- This is a UK based (but international) independent, user-led, organisation established to ensure that all thyroid disease sufferers are given a correct diagnosis and that they receive effective treatment.

Thyroid UK Website: http://www.thyroiduk.org

- This is a thyroid website aimed at providing information and resources to promote effective diagnosis and appropriate treatment for people with thyroid disorders in the UK.

Stop The Thyroid Madness Website: http://www.stopthethyroidmadness.com

- Patient centric website presenting the experience of thyroid patients in an honest and direct way.

Thyroid Patient Forums

- To talk to other thyroid patients about CT3M then join Facebook and search for T3, Recovering with T3 or CT3M. Two Facebook *patient only* groups that may be of value to thyroid patients are:

    https://www.facebook.com/groups/RecoveringWithT3/   and

    https://www.facebook.com/groups/FTPOT3/

Dr. Sarah Myhill's Website: http://www.drmyhill.co.uk/

- Dr. Myhill MB BS currently works full time as a private GP specialising in allergy, nutritional & environmental (ecological) medicine.

Appendix C

A Brief History of Thyroid Testing

OR

Why Do I Feel Like Crap
And Yet All My Blood Tests are Normal?

An Endocrine Patient's Perspective
By
Paul R. Lundy

From the late 1800s until around 1975, doctors were taught how to clinically diagnose thyroid problems by first taking a thorough family history, and then performing a complete physical exam paying attention to any and all signs and symptoms. Because some doctors were more familiar than others in dealing with thyroid problems, the success of the outcome for the patient depended on the skills of their practitioner. Desiccated thyroid was introduced in the mid 1890s, and was used with great success. The standard of treatment was to slowly increase the dose up to the minimum effective dose that relieved the symptoms and left the patient feeling well.

In the 1930s, the Basal Metabolic Rate (BMR) test became the first attempt at a laboratory standard for diagnosing thyroid problems. The BMR checks thyroid function by measuring oxygen consumed when the body is at rest. Unfortunately, it can be complicated to administer and the accuracy was quite often questionable. In the early 1940s, Dr. Broda O. Barnes, M.D., Ph.D., developed the basal temperature test. In August 1942, *The Journal of the American Medical Association* published a study by Dr. Barnes comparing 1,000 college students who had taken both the basal temperature test and the basal metabolic rate test. The study indicated that a low body temperature was a better indication of hypothyroidism than the BMR[1]. Many doctors today still find that the basal temperature test is a useful indicator as a part of the overall picture of the patient's signs and symptoms.

At one point, measuring cholesterol was thought to be an accurate reflection of thyroid status, but that also turned out to be unreliable. Radioactive iodine uptake was another contender, but it too had serious shortcomings. In his book, *Hypothyroidism: The Unsuspected Illness*, Dr. Barnes wrote, "About 1940, the Protein Bound Iodine test for thyroid function came into use. It was to be followed by other laboratory tests to measure thyroid function. For thyroid conditions, the era of the laboratory had appeared. The result was a pendulum-like swing to an extreme. Many physicians came to look upon the results of laboratory tests as absolutes[2]."

For years, physicians had considered a thorough family history along with a complete physical exam, combined with a physician's knowledge of the signs and symptoms of thyroid problems, to be the best approach. Another approach often used by doctors was a short therapeutic trial of desiccated thyroid to see how the patient reacted. With the move to a laboratory standard all you needed was a lab test; the patient, and their signs and symptoms, became somewhat inconsequential.

In April 1965, Dr. Robert D. Utiger, M.D., published his article, "Radioimmunoassay of Human Plasma Thyrotropin", in the *Journal of Clinical Investigation*. Thyrotropin, also known as thyroid-stimulating hormone or TSH, is a glycoprotein hormone synthesized and secreted by the thyrotrope cells in the anterior pituitary gland. It stimulates the thyroid gland to produce more T4 and T3. In the next few years, he and others refined the Thyroid Stimulating Hormone (TSH) test, and Dr. Utiger also developed a serum T3 test. A serum T4 test had already been developed a few years earlier, and had proved unreliable for diagnosing thyroid problems when used alone. Soon the 'Standard Model', an inverse log linear relationship between TSH and T4, which simply means that as TSH goes up then T4 goes down and vice versa, became the accepted model for thyroid feedback and control.

In 1973, a group of leading endocrinologists and thyroidologists, wanting to move to a laboratory standard, made an arbitrary decision to make the TSH test that standard. Within about 2 years, medical schools stopped teaching doctors how to clinically diagnose thyroid problems, and the TSH test soon became widely regarded as the single best test of thyroid function, and still remains so today. If the results of the TSH test are normal, the patient is considered to be euthyroid and no further tests are performed. Performing a TSH test and T4 test together is also common.

There was another consequence to adopting the TSH test as the single diagnostic standard. Because the TSH test was so sensitive to orally given thyroid hormone, it meant that the average dose used before the TSH test was 2 to 3 times greater than the average dose used post TSH test. Dr. David M. Derry, M.D., Ph.D., commented about this in his interview with Mary Shomon[3], and Dr. Denis St. J. O'Reilly, M.D., MSc, wrote about it in his paper, "Thyroid Hormone Replacement: an iatrogenic problem [4]."

Dr. Derry's critique of the TSH test, from the same interview with Mary Shomon, is quite illuminating: "The TSH had a ring of scientific rigor for those who have a smattering of knowledge about thyroid metabolism. It was part of the pituitary feedback mechanism for monitoring the output of the thyroid gland. There is no doubt that it does accomplish this job. But unfortunately the TSH value has no clinical correlation except at absolute extremes with the clinical signs or symptoms of the patient[3]."

In the 1970s and 1980s, synthetic T4 started to replace desiccated thyroid as the treatment of choice. The argument was made that because it was pure it was superior to the desiccated. And, since T4 had a half-life of 7 days compared to the more biologically active T3's half-life, which is usually described as a matter of hours, T4 would provide for a smoother response in the patient. For years the synthetic form suffered from problems with potency and efficacy, and in 1997 the FDA made the manufacturers submit New Drug Applications (NDAs) and demonstrate the stability of the product.

To be fair, Natural Desiccated Thyroid (NDT) was not without its own quality control problems at times either. Although some people seem to do just fine on synthetic T4, there are many of us who do not do well on it at all. There are also some who only do well on T3, although that can be a more complicated solution regarding dosing. Science still does not recognise, nor has it been able to explain thoroughly, why thyroid patients can react so differently to the various thyroid medications.

For years, thyroid patients have been complaining that the TSH test does not seem to match what is going on in our bodies, and that synthetic T4 does not work well for all of us. For years doctors have been ignoring us; we haven't been to medical school. Unless a patient has been randomised, double blinded, and placeboed, we are just anecdotal. As patients, we are often considered incapable of intelligent thought about, or accurate observation of, our own bodies.

At the beginning of the New Millennium, science finally began to catch up to what patients had always known, at least on the testing side. In 2002, a study was published by Anderson et al. in *The Journal of Clinical Endocrinology and Metabolism*[5]. In that study, 16 men were followed for one year measuring TSH, T4, T3, and the free T4 index every month at about the same time. At the end of the year the results were plotted. One individual was excluded because he always had an extremely low TSH. It was found that each individual had a unique thyroid function; that is, each person had their own set point for TSH, T4, and T3, and the set point was slightly different for each person. The range of variation in each individual was actually fairly narrow compared with group reference ranges used to develop laboratory reference ranges. **An individual's range of variation is about half the width of the normal reference range of the TSH test**. The individual range of variation was also narrower for T4, T3 and the free T4 index tests.

"The laboratory reference range is NOT the normal range for an individual[6]."

The reference range is an important part of the TSH test, and the validity of the entire test rests on it. It will determine if you are treated and how you are treated. The sensitivity of the TSH test has improved considerably from the first generation tests, and is now considered sensitive enough for diagnosing hyperthyroidism accurately. This increased sensitivity also helps to improve the accuracy of the reference range, but even with these improvements the reference range is still a problematic area. To understand why, we need to take a closer look at how they are developed.

Dr. Stephanie Lee, M.D., Ph.D., gave a definition of a 'normal range' in her presentation at the 2003 American Thyroid Association (ATA) meeting: "A normal range for any biochemical test is dependent on the assumption that the values of that result, in a normal population, fall in a Gaussian curve and that 95% of 'normals' is two standard deviations on either side of a mean[6]." To establish a group reference range, you usually test 120 or more people who have been rigorously screened for risk factors, and then plot the results and calculate the mean. One standard deviation on either side of the mean accounts for 68% of the set, and two standard deviations on either side accounts for 95% of the set. Another way of looking at it is you take 2½% off the top of the results, and 2½% off the bottom of the results, and this gives you the 95% range of 'normals'. This also means that 5% of the people who are normal are excluded from the normal range.

The bottom of the TSH reference range has been fairly consistent at 0.3 to 0.4 mIU/L. The top end of the range is wider than it should be and is more controversial. If one followed the Gaussian curve, the upper limit would be around 2.5; today however, it is generally around 4.0 to 4.5 mIU/L, unadjusted for age. Just a few years ago the range would have been 0.5 to 5.5, and in previous generations of the test (which were less sensitive) the ranges were higher and even less accurate.

All laboratories establish their own particular reference ranges. If you took a single serum sample and sent it to five different labs, you would likely get five slightly different reference ranges, along with five slightly different results. Age, ethnicity, and geographic location can also affect reference ranges.

"A normal test within the population based laboratory range may not be normal for an individual[6]."

Since the introduction of the TSH test, doctors have treated the laboratory reference range as being equivalent to the patient's reference range, **which it is not**. This has caused problems not only with diagnosing thyroid conditions, but also with treating them. Quite often, a doctor increases a patient's thyroid medication until the TSH test result is in the reference range, and then pronounces the patient fixed. If the patient still complains of symptoms, they are told that since the TSH test is now normal it can't be related to the thyroid and must be something else. Then the patient is usually told that they need to eat better, exercise more, or go see a psychiatrist and get some anti-depressants.

The TSH test is often unreliable if your symptoms are caused by a problem converting T4 to T3, or if you have a high RT3, or you are dealing with other forms of thyroid hormone resistance. Given all the problems we have just looked at, you can begin to understand why the TSH test has been so problematic for so many thyroid patients. This leaves one wondering why it is still the primary diagnostic tool in use today.

In 2002 the National Academy of Clinical Biochemists (NACB) put out new *Laboratory Medicine Practice Guidelines* in which they said: "In the future, it is likely that the upper limit of the serum TSH test euthyroid reference range will be reduced to 2.5 mIU/L because >95% of rigorously screened euthyroid volunteers have serum TSH values between 0.4 and 2.5 mIU/L[7]."

In November 2002, the American Association of Clinical Endocrinologists (AACE) published new treatment guidelines suggesting a range of 0.3 to 3.0. In their January 2003 press release the headline was, "Over 13 million Americans with Thyroid Disease Remain Undiagnosed". The press release goes on to say, "AACE believes the new range will result in proper diagnosis for millions of Americans who suffer from a mild thyroid disorder, but have gone untreated until now[8]." Unfortunately, there are millions of human beings around the planet who are still waiting.

In 2007, a study by Spencer et al. reached this conclusion: "It was hoped that the NHANES III survey would provide definitive TSH reference range data. However, the current analysis shows that an accurate TSH reference range cannot be determined from population data, because occult thyroid dysfunction skews the TSH upper limit. Because of the association of thyroid antibodies with upper TSH values, we believe this dysfunction is related to autoimmune disease, but it may well be due to other unidentified physiological mechanisms[9]." They go on to agree with AACE in using an upper limit of 3.0, and the Endocrine Society in using 2.5 for preconception planning and pregnancy. Then they say this: "These recommendations, however, come with the proviso that sound clinical judgment, based on findings other than TSH concentrations, be exercised with regard to initiating treatment[9]."

For a great many thyroid patients, finding a doctor that is capable of "sound clinical judgment, based on findings other than TSH concentrations" is a difficult task at best. Too many doctors treat the lab test and ignore the patient, along with their signs and symptoms. Quite often we end up having to spend our own money (which is usually not fully reimbursed by insurance) for lab tests and travel to see one of the few doctors actually capable of helping us.

Forty years later, we are still being ruled by the tyranny of the TSH test, which results in an inferior standard of treatment that leaves many of us sick, makes us sicker, or destroys our lives.

For almost 80 years we have been subjected to one testing standard after another. Each was thought to be capable of giving a clear view of what was happening in our bodies, yet all have failed to do so. Serum tests are only clues; they cannot tell us what is happening at the cellular level. There simply is no viable 'one size fits all' approach. Each patient has to figure out what works best in their own body. By sharing the knowledge gained from our collective struggles to regain our lives, we help not only ourselves but others as well. Increasing one's knowledge is the key for a successful outcome, and for becoming an effective advocate for ourselves with the health professionals with whom we work.

June 20, 2013

Appendix D

Adrenal Issues, Testing and CT3M
By
Lynn McGovern

Going on steroids of any kind is a serious decision, whether they are adrenal glandulars or drugs like hydrocortisone (HC). You should not start on any form of steroid replacement unless you have had a minimum of an 8:00 a.m. blood cortisol test, and, preferably, an ACTH stimulation test (also known as a short synacthen test). It is not advisable to use steroids like HC after saliva testing only.

A PROPOSED INITIAL FOCUS ON ADRENAL ISSUES
A good starting point with suspected adrenal issues is to get an adrenal saliva test (AST) done and then to assess the results and see if the AST suggests the presence of adrenal issues. See Chapter 3 of this book for what to look for in AST results.

Adrenal Saliva Tests (ASTs) gather four samples of saliva per day. Only free cortisol passes into saliva, and so an AST is a good way of assessing the overall profile of bio-available cortisol over the day, from morning to evening. When someone gets the AST done, they should ensure that they have all the results for each sample and the reference range for each sample. DHEA results are also helpful. Typically, a good level of cortisol in an AST should have the first sample at the top of the reference range, the second in or near the upper quartile, the third mid-range and the fourth at the low end of the reference range.

CT3M is often a good solution for dealing with low cortisol, and thyroid patients may wish to start with this first.

BEFORE CONSIDERING THE USE OF HC
Before ever considering the use of HC, it is advisable to consider the following:

- CT3M. It is sensible to give the CT3M time to work before considering adrenal hormone replacement. Trying CT3M for a week and then giving up would be a useless endeavour. It takes time to implement CT3M and you need to allow the adrenals time to respond.

- Testing for iron deficiency. Low levels of iron can cause symptoms such as heart palpitations and fatigue. Such symptoms may mimic adrenal insufficiency. Make sure that you get a full iron panel, including transferrin saturation percentage, total iron binding capacity (TIBC), serum iron and serum ferritin.

- Testing sex hormones. Low sex hormones can cause symptoms that may also mimic adrenal insufficiency, so it is important to get these tested and optimised. For further help on this issue see a qualified and experienced doctor or consider joining the Sexy Hormones Facebook Group: https://www.facebook.com/groups/sexyhormones/.

- Testing for B12 and folate deficiency. Low levels of these important nutrients can mimic hypothyroidism and weaken adrenal function.

OTHER NON-STEROID OPTIONS FOR THE ADRENALS

Adaptogenic herbs – Liquorice root works to extend the half-life of cortisol, keeping it longer in the body. However, it does not actually increase cortisol. Other adaptogenic herbs may help, such as Rhodiola and Holy Basil. Please see Chapter 10 of this book for more information on adaptogens. This paper also has a lot of comprehensive information on herbs: http://www.healingpoints.com/Adrenal.PDF.

Low Dose Naltrexone (LDN) has really helped some patients improve their cortisol response. This may be due to the effect of increased endorphins on the HPA axis (hypothalamic pituitary axis) leading to more ACTH and therefore more cortisol output. However, this is just speculation. For some, LDN is a great option to try if CT3M has not done enough on its own. Please see Chapter 20 of this book for more information on LDN.

WHAT IF CT3M FAILS TO ADDRESS THE ADRENAL ISSUE?

CT3M takes some time to work, and it is well worth continuing with this, and perhaps enhancing its use by adding in either LDN or adaptogens (or both) before beginning to look at further testing.

If adrenal insufficiency continues to be a significant problem after CT3M has been tried for an adequate period of time, or if the symptoms are very severe, then a number of comprehensive laboratory tests should be performed before beginning medically supervised treatment with a steroid like HC. This is because many doctors who prescribe HC without these tests do so with the expectation that their patient will be able to wean off. If the patient cannot wean, and they actually have some form of permanent adrenal problem (which cannot be diagnosed now without weaning off HC and becoming very ill), they will be in serious trouble, badly needing steroids to function, but without a doctor to write the prescription. In the most extreme of cases, withdrawing from much needed steroids can be fatal. Dex (dexamethasone), is sometimes used as an alternative to HC. Dex is a long acting, more potent steroid than hydrocortisone.

There is also always a danger of adrenal suppression when taking HC or any other steroids. This means, that even if the adrenals worked beforehand, they may atrophy (shrink) after a certain amount of time on steroids and may never work properly again. Patients will also require more steroids at certain times, such as pregnancy or illness. Without an official diagnosis, extra steroids can be hard to source.

The following are established adrenal diagnoses:
- Congenital adrenal hyperplasia (CAH) - This is a genetic mutation involving a defect in the enzymes needed to produce cortisol. As a result, the adrenal glands are constantly stimulated in a desperate attempt to make cortisol. Since the adrenal glands also make

androgens, this can results in large amounts of testosterone going into the bloodstream. This disorder is almost always diagnosed at birth as it results in virilisation (masculinisation) of female genitals.
http://www.endocrineonline.org/pdf%20box/cah.pdf

- Late-onset congenital adrenal hyperplasia (LOCAH) - This is a type of CAH that presents anytime from early childhood to early adulthood. Genitals appear normal at birth with this condition, but the person generally encounters problems during puberty. LOCAH is often misdiagnosed as PCOS, as it has very similar symptoms. http://www.caresfoundation.org/productcart/pc/ncah_late_onset_cah.html

- Cushing's syndrome – This is a disorder caused by prolonged exposure to high levels of cortisol. It is generally caused by a tumour of some kind or by long-term usage of very high dose steroids. There is also a form of Cushing's called cyclical Cushing's that causes a person to swing from high levels of cortisol to normal levels of cortisol. http://www.nlm.nih.gov/medlineplus/ency/article/000348.htm

- Addison's disease/primary adrenal insufficiency - Addison's disease is an autoimmune disease that causes the gradual destruction of the adrenal glands. This results in low levels of cortisol. http://www.nlm.nih.gov/medlineplus/ency/article/000378.htm

- Secondary adrenal insufficiency - This is a disorder whereby the body cannot make enough ACTH. The body needs ACTH to stimulate the adrenal glands to make cortisol. So, the adrenals themselves may be working fine, but the pituitary cannot signal the adrenal glands to produce the correct amounts of cortisol. Secondary adrenal insufficiency is said to be more common than primary adrenal insufficiency.

- Partial adrenal insufficiency -This is a type of adrenal disorder whereby the adrenals sometimes make enough cortisol and sometimes not. Many people refer to this condition as "adrenal fatigue". "Partial adrenal insufficiency" is however the more correct medical term. http://www.goodhormonehealth.com/adrenal-cecils.pdf

COMPREHENSIVE ADRENAL TESTING (if CT3M is not working well enough)

The following can affect cortisol testing: steroid medications, steroid creams, steroid sprays, Florinef, adrenal glandulars, adaptogenic herbs, inositol, 5-HTP, PABA, GABA, natural progesterone, melatonin, cordyceps, theanine, caffeine, zinc, magnolia root extract, DHEA, anti-depressants, sleeping pills, benzodiazepines such as xanax, beta blockers, asthma medications, blood pressure medications, Imitrex, beta blockers and medications for AHDD. Hydrocortisone cream can also affect the tests. Therefore, it is important to avoid these before doing any of the tests below. There is no straight answer available as to when to come off these before testing. However, it has been suggested that the HPA axis can take up to two years to return to what it was prior to steroid usage - hence why testing must be done before steroid use. Adaptogenic herbs and glandulars do not tend to suppress the HPA axis in the same way, so usually a month off them should be okay. It is recommended that that a person should be off anti-depressants for six weeks before testing.

A morning blood cortisol at 8 a.m. This test needs to be performed as close to 8 a.m. as possible. This is because the ideal morning cortisol ranges are based on this time. Doing the test at noon may give some useful information, but it likely will not help get an official diagnosis of adrenal insufficiency. Please see the following paper for optimal cortisol levels: http://dspace.dial.pipex.com/town/estate/aquc35/book/adrenal.pdf. Divide the figures by 27.6 to get US units. The UK typically uses nmol/L as their cortisol measuring unit, while the US uses µg/dl as their unit. So 300 nmol/L would be 10.6 µg/dl in US units. You can also use this calculator to convert units: http://www.endmemo.com/medical/unitconvert/Estradiol.php. **Here is an explanation of various a.m. cortisol levels:**

- Definitive adrenal insufficiency: < 6 ug/dl (< 165 nmol/L)
- Very low cortisol levels: < 11 ug/dl (< 300 nmol/L)
- Sub-optimal cortisol levels: < 18 ug/dl (< 496.8 nmol/L)

An ACTH short synacthen test (also known as a STIM test). An ACTH stimulation test measures the maximum quantity of cortisol that the adrenal glands can produce, and as such, is the best way of identifying disease of the adrenal glands themselves. It is also the only officially recognised diagnostic test. However, it must be done between the hours of 8-9 a.m., since all the ideal results are based on morning readings. Do not submit to an ACTH STIM test in the afternoon, as results may not be accurate. An ACTH STIM test involves drawing a baseline cortisol (same as the a.m. cortisol listed above) and then drawing further blood cortisols at 30 minutes and sixty minutes. It also involves drawing a baseline ACTH. The following is useful in the interpretation of ACTH STIM test results:

- In her paper, Dr Arlt notes that adrenal insufficiency can be excluded if a person has a peak 60 minute cortisol of > 21.7 µg/dl (> 600 nmol/L).
- However, many patient advocates state that an optimal result on this test is actually at least 30 µg/dl (828 nmol/L).

An ACTH blood test. An ACTH blood test is not enough information on its own; however it is useful in combination with an ACTH STIM Test or a.m. cortisol testing. Low in range or under-range ACTH in combination with low cortisol would indicate secondary adrenal insufficiency, whereas high in range or over-range ACTH in combination with low cortisol would indicate primary adrenal insufficiency. Please note that ACTH specimens are highly sensitive and need to be stored on ice. Improper storage of ACTH specimens can invalidate the test.

Insulin Tolerance Test. If you suspect you have secondary adrenal insufficiency, you may need to get an ITT. This involves being injected with insulin to lower your blood sugar. Then, once your blood sugar is low, cortisol levels are measured. Cortisol levels should be normal-high when a person has low blood sugar. If they remain low even during hypoglycaemia, this shows that there is a problem with the HPA axis. In order for the test to be valid, your blood sugar must plummet to 39.6 mg/dl (2.2 nmol/L). See: http://www.pathology.leedsth.nhs.uk/dnn_bilm/Investigationprotocols/Pituitaryprotocols/InsulinToleranceTest.aspx

Cortisol saliva testing (also known as an adrenal stress test or AST). This test is most useful if the other tests appear "normal". However if the blood cortisol is low then there is no real need to get this test. It is important to look at the total daily cortisol level as well as each of the four samples.

Cortisol Binding Globulin. This is a new test that is not on most doctors' radar, whether they are endocrinologists, naturopaths or GPs. However, it can be a very illuminating test. Cortisol binding globulin (CBG) is a binding protein that binds up cortisol. The more CBG a person has in their system, the less cortisol they have free to do its job. So a person could have a perfect morning cortisol of 20 µg/dl (552 nmol/L), yet all of this cortisol could be bound up by high amounts of CBG. Please see the following links:
http://www.ncbi.nlm.nih.gov/pubmed/11834433 and http://www.endocrine-abstracts.org/ea/0003/ea0003p243.htm

Please remember that you must always work with a doctor in order to get a diagnosis and treatment.

So, unless cortisol meets criteria for definitive adrenal insufficiency, the circadian T3 method (CT3M)) may well help struggling adrenal performance. The strategies outlined in the Recovering with T3 book and The CT3M Handbook may be sufficient to restore excellent adrenal health. If you have tried CT3M for a good period of time, and are still very ill, then comprehensive adrenal tests above should definitely be performed.

WHAT TO DO WITH RESULTS OF COMPREHENSIVE ADRENAL TESTING
What you do next depends on whether:
1) The cortisol results are SUB-OPTIMAL OR
2) The cortisol results are VERY LOW and you have already tried CT3M without a good enough response OR
3) The cortisol results meet the criteria for definitive adrenal insufficiency

Let me deal with each of these cases separately.

Sub-Optimal or Very Low Results. CT3M can often be of benefit in these cases and so we suggest trying CT3M first.

We would expect someone to experience at least some benefit from CT3M within three months or less. This might not be enough for someone to feel well, but, if there is some improvement, then it is worth titrating the circadian and other doses to see if more can be achieved. If it becomes clear that little or no further improvement is likely and there is still not enough cortisol being produced, then we would suggest using additional or alternative approaches, e.g. adaptogenic herbs or LDN. Adrenal glandulars could also be considered at some point. If none of these have helped, then the individual may be able to add some small doses of HC at the times of day where their cortisol is low, along with continuing with CT3M. This would need to be done under medical supervision.

Unfortunately, the HPA axis is exquisitely sensitive, so even small amounts of HC can shut it down. If the feedback loop is shut down by your taking HC, this means that your body has shut down what little cortisol it used to produce, so you could actually end up with less cortisol than you started with. Some people are lucky enough to not have this happen, but many find this is a problem when taking more than 5 mg HC. Even as little as 10 mg HC can shut down the feedback loop. Therefore, if the goal is to not be dependent on steroids, it would be prudent to start with less than 10 mg HC per day.

Definitive Adrenal Insufficiency. If the results indicate that replacement cortisol is the route to go (an a.m. cortisol of < 6 µg/dl (< 165 nmol/L) OR a STIM result of < 21.7 µg/dl (< 600 nmol/L), it is important that you begin a physiological dosing regimen. An a.m. cortisol of < 6 µg/dl (< 165 nmol/L) is technically enough for a diagnosis of definitive adrenal insufficiency; however most doctors will insist on performing a ACTH STIM test, no matter how low the a.m. cortisol result is.

Before submitting to HC only however, we recommend combining HC with CT3M, as many have found this reduces their steroid needs. For example, if CT3M has helped (but just not enough), then CT3M can be combined with a small amount of additional cortisol, perhaps up to 10 mg of HC per day in divided doses. A sign (lowering of temp at a specific time) that correlates to the adrenal saliva test (low cortisol) would be a clue as to when to add the HC. For example: Temp drops at 11:30 a.m. and fatigue ensues, while the cortisol test shows that cortisol is low at noon. HC could be introduced at 10:30 a.m. at 2.5 mg. Then some days could be left for observation to see if the person improves. If there is no improvement, then the HC dose could be increased from 2.5 mg HC to 5 mg. If the person needs a second dose, then this could start at 2.5 mg 3-4 hours after the first dose, or even later if symptoms indicate. Eventually, if adrenal health continues to improve over time, the person may need to lower and eventually discontinue their use of HC. This would need to be done in combination with a doctor and with the use of thorough adrenal testing, however. Nobody should ever just abruptly stop their usage of HC.

Please be advised that the dosage level for people not doing CT3M, but who work full-time, are on thyroid medicines and who wish to exercise tends to be 25-40 mg HC. Some people can get by on 20 mg of HC, but these people aren't usually on thyroid medicines, and don't usually work full time or wish to follow an exercise regime.

Typical uses of HC involve starting at least an hour before rising, at lunchtime and then late afternoon. HC is not usually taken later than 5:00 p.m. unless the person has to go to bed very late (a few people need to take a small amount of HC at bed-time).

THE FOLLOWING ARE PATIENT BASED ADRENAL SUPPORT GROUPS:
Addison's support group: http://www.addisonssupport.com
FTPO Adrenals: https://www.facebook.com/groups/FTPOAdrenals

LINKS:
Dr Arlt paper: http://dspace.dial.pipex.com/town/estate/aquc35/book/adrenal.pdf
Dr Friedman's paper on partial adrenal insufficiency:
http://www.goodhormonehealth.com/adrenal-cecils.pdf
Cortisol saliva is a measure of free cortisol throughout the day:
http://www.sciencedirect.com/science/article/pii/0009898181903533
Unit calculator: http://www.endmemo.com/medical/unitconvert/Estradiol.php

Appendix E

References By Chapter

Chapter 1

1. Robinson, P.: *Recovering with T3 My Journey from Hypothyroidism to Good Health Using the T3 Thyroid Hormone.* Elephant in the Room Books. Revised Edition 2013.
2. Russell, W., Harrison, R.F., Smith, N., Darzy, K., Shalet, S., Weetman, A.P., Ross, R.J.: Free triiodothyronine has a distinct circadian rhythm that is delayed but parallels thyrotropin levels. *J Clin Endocrinol Metab.* 93(6):2300-6. June 2008. Abstract may be found at: http://jcem.endojournals.org/content/93/6/2300.
3. Robinson, P.: RecoveringwithT3.com. Success Stories. <http://recoveringwitht3.com/success_story>

Chapter 2

1. Russell, W., Harrison, R.F., Smith, N., Darzy, K., Shalet, S., Weetman, A.P., Ross, R.J.: Free triiodothyronine has a distinct circadian rhythm that is delayed but parallels thyrotropin levels. *J Clin Endocrinol Metab.* 93(6):2300-6. June 2008. Abstract may be found at: http://jcem.endojournals.org/content/93/6/2300.
2. Dietrich, J.W., Landgrafe, G., Fotiadou, E.H.: TSH and Thyrotropic Agonists: Key Actors in Thyroid Homeostatis. *Journal of Thyroid Research.* Volume 2012(2012), Article ID 351864, doi:10.1155/2012/351864.
3. Conti, A., Studer, H., Kneubuehl, F., Kohler, H.: Regulation of Thyroidal Deiodinase Activity. *Endocrinology,* Vol. 102 (1):321-329, 1978.
4. Ikeda, K., Takeuchi, T., Ito, Y., Murakami, I., Mokuda, O., Tominaga, M., Mashiba, H.: Effect of thyrotropin on conversion of T4 to T3 in perfused rat liver. *Life Sciences,* Volume 38, Issue 20:1801-1806, 1986.
5. Ikeda, T., Honda M., Murakami, I., Kuno, S., Mokuda, O., Tokumori, Y., Tominaga, M., Mashiba, H.: Effect of TSH on conversion of T4 to T3 in perfused rat kidney. *Metabolism,* Volume 34, Issue 11:1057-1060, 1985.
6. Robinson, P.: *Recovering with T3 My Journey from Hypothyroidism to Good Health Using the T3 Thyroid Hormone.* Elephant in the Room Books. Revised Edition 2013. Chapters, 16, 25.
7. Robinson, P.: *Recovering with T3 My Journey from Hypothyroidism to Good Health Using the T3 Thyroid Hormone.* Elephant in the Room Books. Revised Edition 2013. Chapter 12.
8. Robinson, P.: *Recovering with T3 My Journey from Hypothyroidism to Good Health Using the T3 Thyroid Hormone.* Elephant in the Room Books. Revised Edition 2013. Chapter 2.
9. Escobar-Morreale, H.F., Obregon, M.J., del Rey, F.E., de Escobar, G.M.: Only the Combined Treatment with Thyroxine and Triiodothyronine Ensures Euthyroidism in All Tissues. *Endocrinology,* 137(6):2490-2502, 1996.
10. Robinson, P.: Why The Circadian T3 Method is So Important. September 2013. *Recovering with T3 Website.* <http://recoveringwitht3.com/blog/why-circadian-t3-method-so-important>

Chapter 3

1. Robinson, P.: *Recovering with T3 My Journey from Hypothyroidism to Good Health Using the T3 Thyroid Hormone.* Elephant in the Room Books. Revised Edition 2013. Chapter 3, 'Adrenal Insufficiency' sub-section.
2. Robinson, P.: *Recovering with T3 My Journey from Hypothyroidism to Good Health Using the T3 Thyroid Hormone.* Elephant in the Room Books. Revised Edition 2013. Chapter 4, 'Iron' sub-section.
3. Bowthorpe, J.A.: Stop the Thyroid Madness website. Iron information. http://www.stopthethyroidmadness.com/ferritin/
4. Bowthorpe, J.A.: *Stop the Thyroid Madness.* Laughing Grape Publishing, 2008.
5. Robinson, P.: *Recovering with T3 My Journey from Hypothyroidism to Good Health Using the T3 Thyroid Hormone.* Elephant in the Room Books. Revised Edition 2013. Chapter 4, 'B12', 'Folic Acid' and 'Vitamin D' sub-sections.
6. Robinson, P.: *Recovering with T3 My Journey from Hypothyroidism to Good Health Using the T3 Thyroid Hormone.* Elephant in the Room Books. Revised Edition 2013. Chapter 5, 'Interaction with Sex Hormones' sub-section'.

Chapter 5

1. Robinson, P.: *Recovering with T3 My Journey from Hypothyroidism to Good Health Using the T3 Thyroid Hormone.* Elephant in the Room Books. Revised Edition 2013. Chapter 14, 'Lesson #7 Waves of T3' sub-section.

Chapter 6

1. Robinson, P.: *Recovering with T3 My Journey from Hypothyroidism to Good Health Using the T3 Thyroid Hormone.* Elephant in the Room Books. Revised Edition 2013. Chapters 4, 19.

Chapter 7

1. Robinson, P.: *Recovering with T3 My Journey from Hypothyroidism to Good Health Using the T3 Thyroid Hormone.* Elephant in the Room Books. Revised Edition 2013. Chapter 5, 'Blood Sugar Balance' sub-section.

Chapter 8

1. Robinson, P.: *Recovering with T3 My Journey from Hypothyroidism to Good Health Using the T3 Thyroid Hormone.* Elephant in the Room Books. Revised Edition 2013. Chapter 4, 'Iron' sub-section.
2. Robinson, P.: *Recovering with T3 My Journey from Hypothyroidism to Good Health Using the T3 Thyroid Hormone.* Elephant in the Room Books. Revised Edition 2013. Chapter 4.
3. Brownstein, D.: *Iodine Why You Need It.* Third Edition. Alternative Medical Press. 2008.
4. Robinson, P.: Calming the Autoantibody Attack in Hashimoto's Thyroiditis. October 2012. *Recovering with T3 Website.* <http://recoveringwitht3.com/blog/calming-autoantibody-attack-hashimotos-thyroiditis>
5. Robinson, P.: *Recovering with T3 My Journey from Hypothyroidism to Good Health Using the T3 Thyroid Hormone.* Elephant in the Room Books. Revised Edition 2013. Chapter 5, 'Blood Sugar Balance' sub-section.
6. Robinson, P.: *Recovering with T3 My Journey from Hypothyroidism to Good Health Using the T3 Thyroid Hormone.* Elephant in the Room Books. Revised Edition 2013. Chapter 5, 'Environmental Toxins' sub-section.
7. Cutler, A. H.: *Amalgam Illness: Diagnosis & Treatment: What You Can Do to Get Better, How Your Doctor Can Help You.* 1999.
8. Robinson, P.: *Recovering with T3 My Journey from Hypothyroidism to Good Health Using the T3 Thyroid Hormone.* Elephant in the Room Books. Revised Edition 2013. Chapter 5, 'Interaction with Sex Hormones' sub-section'.
9. Ladose Withrawal. *Point of Return Website.* <http://www.pointofreturn.com/ladose_withdrawal.html>
10. Manthey, L., Leeds, C., Giltay, E.J., van Teen, T., Vreeburg, S.A., Penninx, B.W., Zitman, F.G.: Antidepressant use and salivary cortisol in depressive and anxiety disorders. *Eur Neuropsychopharmacol.* 2011. Sep; 21(9):691-9. See abstract on <http://www.ncbi.nlm.nih.gov/pubmed/21458959>
11. Kharrazian, D.: *Why Do I Still Have Thyroid Symptoms? When My Lab Tests Are Normal.* New York, Morgan James Publishing, 2010.
12. Campbell McBride, N.: *Gut and Psychology Syndrome.* MedInform Publishing. 2010.
13. Davis, W.: *Wheat Belly.* Rodale. 2011.
14. Braly, J., Hoggan, R.: *Dangerous Grains.* Avery Health Guides. 2003.
15. Wangen, S.: *Healthier Without Wheat.* Innate Health Publishing. 2009.

16. Sanfilippo, D.: *Practical Paleo: A Customized Approach to Health and Whole-Foods Lifestyle.* Victory Belt Publishing. 2012.
17. Robinson, P.: *Recovering with T3 My Journey from Hypothyroidism to Good Health Using the T3 Thyroid Hormone.* Elephant in the Room Books. Revised Edition 2013. Chapters 4, 5, 29.

Chapter 13

1. Robinson, P.: *Recovering with T3 My Journey from Hypothyroidism to Good Health Using the T3 Thyroid Hormone.* Elephant in the Room Books. Revised Edition 2013. Chapter 14, 'Lesson #7 Waves of T3' sub-section.

Chapter 14

1. Robinson, P.: *Recovering with T3 My Journey from Hypothyroidism to Good Health Using the T3 Thyroid Hormone.* Elephant in the Room Books. Revised Edition 2013. Chapter 16, 'Time When Majority of Cortisol is Produced' sub-section.

Chapter 16

1. Robinson, P.: *Recovering with T3 My Journey from Hypothyroidism to Good Health Using the T3 Thyroid Hormone.* Elephant in the Room Books. Revised Edition 2013. Chapters 21, 22, 23.
2. Robinson, P.: *Recovering with T3 My Journey from Hypothyroidism to Good Health Using the T3 Thyroid Hormone.* Elephant in the Room Books. Revised Edition 2013. Chapter 22.

Appendix C

1. Dr. Broda O. Barnes Hypothyroidism: The Unsuspected Illness P 43.
2. Dr. Broda O. Barnes Hypothyroidism: The Unsuspected Illness P 136.
3. Mary Shomon interviews Dr. David Derry, M.D., Ph.D. Re: TSH Tests http://thyroid.about.com/od/thyroiddrugtreatments/l/blderryb.htm
4. Dr. Denis St J. O'Reilly, Thyroid Hormone Replacement: an iatrogenic problem. Int J Clin Pract, June 2010, 64, 7, 991-994.
5. Andersen S, Pedersen KM, Bruun NH, Laurberg P. Narrow individual variations in serum T(4) and T(3) in normal subjects: a clue to the understanding of subclinical thyroid disease. J Clin Endocrinol Metab. 2002 87: 1068-1072.
6. Dr. Stephanie Lee, M.D., Ph.D., TSH Reference Range Redefined: What does it Mean and What Should We Do? American Thyroid Association 2003, 75th Annual Meeting, http://site.blueskybroadcast.com/Client/P3/
7. The National Academy of Clinical Biochemistry Presents Laboratory Medicine Practice Guidelines, Volume 13/2002, P 34.
8. American Association of Clinical Endocrinologists, Press Release, January 2003, 'Over 13 Million Americans With Thyroid Disease Remain Undiagnosed', Retrieved from, http://www.hospitalsoup.com/public/AACEPress_release-highlighted.pdf
9. Spencer C, Hollowell J, Kazarosyan M, Braverman L, National Health and Nutrition Examination Survey III Thyroid-Stimulating Hormone (TSH)-Thyroperoxidase Antibody Relationships Demonstrate That TSH Upper Reference Limits May Be Skewed By Occult Thyroid Dysfunction, JCEM 92(11):4326-42

Index

CPSIA information can be obtained
at www.ICGtesting.com
Printed in the USA
BVOW07s1234291016

466053BV00012B/59/P